the SMART WEIGH

the

SMART
WEIGH

The Simple, New 5-Point Plan
for Losing Weight Forever—
Without Losing Your Soul

PAMELA M. SMITH, R.D.

LifeLine
Press

A Regnery Publishing Company
Washington, D.C.

Library of Congress Cataloging-in-Publication Data
on file with the Library of Congress.

Published in the United States by
LifeLine Press
A Regnery Publishing Company
One Massachusetts Avenue, NW
Washington, DC 20001

Visit us at www.lifelinepress.com

Distributed to the trade by
National Book Network
4720-A Boston Way
Lanham, MD 20706

Printed on acid-free paper
Manufactured in the United States of America

10 9 8 7 6 5 4 3 2 1

Books are available in quantity for promotional or premium use. Write to Director of Special Sales, Regnery Publishing, Inc., One Massachusetts Avenue, NW, Washington, DC 20001, for information on discounts and terms, or call (202) 216-0600.

TO LARRY, DANIELLE, AND NICOLE...
Loving you is food to my soul.

CONTENTS

Acknowledgement

I am forever grateful to so many people who have made The Smart Weigh a living reality:

Special thanks to those at LifeLine Press—Jeff Carneal, Marji Ross, Karen Anderson, Mike Ward, Molly Mullen, and Lauren Lawson—for investing their incredible gifts and talents into bringing this message forth and propelling it forward, and to Jack Croft, who so skillfully worked as a master sculptor.

To my loving family—especially my Mom—for faithfully being my best cheerleaders and replenishers.

And to all my awesome clients. Your life experiences—your hurdles and your victories—have shaped The Smart Weigh. Thank you for choosing a way of life—not just another diet. May you be ever filled with great food and great health—and energy for life!

PART 1

GET SMART, LOSE WEIGHT

CHAPTER 1

LEARNING TO LIVE THE SMART WEIGH

FOR TWO DECADES NOW, I've coached thousands of people who have come to my nutrition practice wanting to lose weight, gain energy, and recapture the joy of living. Almost every one had been on at least one fad diet or another over the years. They would lose weight, only to eventually regain every pound—and then some. When they arrived at my office for the first time, they were overweight, tired, and stressed.

I knew just how they felt. It was like looking in a mirror at my own past.

Like many of you, I grew up with dieting as my second language— a bona fide member of the Dieting Generation. And with good reason: I inherited a tendency toward being overweight and had a family filled with compulsive overeaters and obesity. By the time I was eleven I had already gone on my first diet, an awful grapefruit and poached egg diet. Was I overweight at the time? Not really. But I was growing and at the start of menses, and my body shape was changing. My hips simply didn't conform to the popular "Twiggy" look of the day. Add to that an unhealthy dose of fear about my family's obesity problems, and I became a charter member of the Dieting Generation.

I lost weight at first. But, sadly, I regained it—more than I had lost. It was the classic story: I lost five pounds only to gain that five and raise it three. The next year, on the next diet (five days of spinach and orange juice!), I lost ten pounds, and quite quickly gained fifteen. The pendulum was swinging higher and wider each year with each new diet. All the dieting was doing was leaving me a malnourished mess, yet weighing more and more. I spent half my time discouraged and depressed—and the other half overeating to compensate.

In the last semester of my senior year at Florida State University, I got a wake-up call. I was anxious to graduate and take on the world of fashion design and marketing. I needed a class to fill a core requirement for my chosen field and stumbled on a class in nutrition. I was on one of my many diets at the time—lose-five-pounds-in-five-days-for-a-weekend-beach-party crash diet. It was straight out of the newest diet book on the block, *Dr. Atkins' Diet Revolution*, and it was working great! I had actually shown a loss of twelve pounds in seven days! It was miraculous... and definitely the way I was going to eat for the rest of my life.

But then, sitting in this nutrition class in the early seventies, I was amazed to learn of the damage I was doing to my body by following this diet and all the others, by my naiveté and drive for thinness at any cost. And, like all crash dieters, I was paying a high price: poor health, mood swings, and a body that was yo-yoing between fat and lean. I was an "expert" dieter, but I didn't have a clue what I was doing. While taking the course, I began to understand that I knew precious little about health. I had not been taught, I had only been mentored by diet doctors and gurus who had become successful by selling quick ways to lose weight, not giving the full story about caring for the whole body.

After an emotional seesaw and much deliberation, I changed my major to nutrition. It was the first thing in my life that I really felt

---

WARNING SIGNS OF A BAD DIET

1. Forbidden Foods. Any diet that restricts or cuts out whole food groups is guaranteed to cause problems. Not only will the deprivation lead to binges; it cuts out exposure to essential nutrients and nutriceuticals (pharmacological agents in food that are vital for vibrant living). Although choices need to be made wisely, all types of real food fit into a healthy diet.

2. Very Low Calories. A normally active woman trying to lose weight should consume no fewer than 1,500 calories per day. A normally active man trying to lose weight should consume no fewer than 1,800 calories per day.

3. Speedy Results. For healthy, permanent weight loss, you should aim to lose no more than one to two pounds per week.

4. No Exercise. A healthy weight loss plan should encourage at least thirty minutes of moderate-intensity exercise four to five days per week.

5. Infrequent Meals. It's best to eat before you get intensely hungry. For most people, that's at least every three to four hours.

---

passionate about—I had to help others learn what I was learning and break free from the vicious dieting cycle right along with me. That decision changed my life—and changed my dieting ways. I never went on a diet again.

Discovering The Smart Weigh

As I learned more about nutrition and began to take care of my body, I was able to lose weight and, for the first time, gain health and energy. My nails became strong and long, my hair was shiny and full, my eyes were clear and sparkling. I no longer got headaches every day, nor did I sit on the cliff of depression. I could think clearly—even studying was less of a chore. I grew in understanding of why I did what I did, and why I didn't do the things I wanted to do when it came to self-care and healthy eating.

I have now been living this life of wellness and teaching it for twenty-two years. Throughout my years of nutritional and behavioral counseling, people have come to me seeking a quality of life filled with energy and well-being. Many people have knocked on my door because they want to lose weight for good. Some need to manage stress better. Some want more energy. Others arrive very ill, in need of a nutritional plan to control serious disease—even to save their lives.

I started my nutrition practice as a Registered Dietitian for a progressive hospital's oncology unit, working with very brave patients and their families to fight their cancer with every means available. These challenging days led me into private practice working with people seeking wellness, helping them to get well and live well today, while focusing on preventing the diseases of tomorrow.

Early in my practice I sensed that, like my dieting college self, most of my clients needed simple nutritional education and guidance. They needed to be led beyond the cultural diet deceptions and myths to a true understanding of holistic health and nutrition. Rather than finding out what they shouldn't eat, they needed to learn what they should eat, when to eat, and how to balance their intake in a way that would benefit their bodies. My clients needed to learn how to break away from the typical American eating style while still living a normal lifestyle. And they needed to learn the vital part food plays in their well-being.

Different from the run-of-the-mill physicians and programs, I worked with my clients in a very focused, time-intensive manner. The foundation of their lifestyle changes was individual and practical. In 1985 I developed The Smart Weigh, a seven-week plan of practical education and lifestyle direction. Since then, more than 12,000 people have followed the program. And now you can, too.

Like my clients, you'll discover that the best diet is one that focuses on real foods that you like and can live with, one that is generous in complex carbohydrates, moderate in lean proteins, and light on fat. One that calls for eating small, balanced meal portions often throughout the day, drinking water, and moderate exercise.

Unlike the diet designers you may have followed or been taught by in the past, I emphasize eating, not starving or manipulating the body. The emphasis is not just on what to eat, but on how and when to best stabilize body chemistries, boost the metabolic burn, handle stress, and release your full energy. The Smart Weigh is a week-by-week building plan that enables you to function close to your peak in seven weeks: thinner, more fit, and equipped to continue on that positive road to your goals—for life.

Remember this: You don't need to learn how to diet; you need to learn how to eat in a healthy way. The strategies in the pages that follow will change your perspective about the place of food, exercise, and rest in your life, and they will greatly enhance your understanding of your body.

You can take charge, feel better, have abundant energy from morning till night, and look more radiant and healthy. Forget the "miracles." Save your money, your time, and maybe even your life—do it The Smart Weigh.

The Three Keys to Permanent Weight Loss

Weight gain is not inevitable for men or women—nor is it inevitable if you have a genetic proclivity. If you have been gaining weight—or been unable to lose it—it's probably because your fat cells are responding in survival mode. Fighting them with a fad diet only locks them into metabolic slowdown. That's why the only way to manage weight permanently is to forego dieting and begin to live in a new and natural way that unlocks the exit door to your fat cells so they can start releasing fat again.

Getting your body working for you and shedding excess pounds is within your control. First, you need to understand the three keys to permanent weight loss. These keys are the foundation upon which The Smart Weigh is built. Cracking the fat cell code and living The Smart Weigh begins with choosing a way of eating and living that is so comfortable that you can live with it the rest of your life.

1. Stoke Your Metabolic Fire

It's not the calories taken in but the calories burned that count—and your metabolism makes all the difference. Your metabolism is the chemical process that converts food to energy and is measured by how many calories you burn per minute for body functions—both voluntary movement, and automatic, involuntary functions like breathing, heart beat, digestion, and blood circulation. The greatest amount of calories used (70 percent) are those burned to maintain this basic body function.

At a cellular level, our metabolism is activated by a balance of supply and demand: a supply of optimum fuel and oxygen to the cells for energy metabolism, and a demand from the body systems for energy. A combination of factors—especially our stressful lifestyles and lack of self-care—causes our fat cells to lock down, slowing our metabolic rate to a snail's pace, which results in fats being stored rather than burned for energy. Although a calorie is a calorie, your metabolism can increase or decrease (burn or store those calories) depending on your eating patterns. The body was designed to slow itself down to protect against energy deficits. As a result, erratic eating patterns keep our metabolism locked in low gear, storing away every meal as if it were our last.

Think of your metabolism as a campfire that requires fuel to burn, and air to fan the fire's flame. A campfire dies down during the night and must have wood added in the morning to begin to burn brightly once more. Without being "stoked" with new fuel, the spark turns to ash—there's nothing left to burn.

Similarly, your body awakens in a slowed-down state. If you don't "break the fast" with breakfast and continue to feed it through the day to meet your body's demand for energy and boost your metabolic system, your body turns to its own muscle mass (not fat) for energy and slows down even more, conserving itself for a potentially long, starved state. Then, when the evening eating begins, most of that food will be stored as fat because the body isn't burning energy at a fast rate; the fire has gone out. The food you eat, after long hours without, is like an armload of firewood being dumped on a dead fire.

Regardless of the number of calories consumed when we do eat, the body can use only a small amount of energy, protein, and other nutrients quickly. The rest is thrown off as waste or stored as fat. Eating the American way robs the body of vital nutrients for the remaining twenty-four hours—until the next feeding frenzy. We not only go wrong in how much we eat or what we eat, we also eat entirely too much at the wrong time. Most of us get most of our calories after 6 P.M.—much too late.

Life in the Fast Food Lane

To burn the calories you consume—to metabolize them into energy, rather than store them as fat—requires nutrients. These vital nutrients are the vitamins, minerals, and phytochemicals found in foods. Certain nutrients are considered essential for the metabolism because they act as catalysts for calorie burning. The B-complex vitamins, magnesium, and zinc are important examples. (We'll talk more about them in Chapter 3.) Also important is chromium, found in whole grains, which helps to transport glucose through the cell membranes so that it can be burned for energy. Iron is also vital because it delivers oxygen inside the cells, "fanning the flame" of calorie burning.

Many people may be getting plenty of calories, but not enough of the nutrients to help metabolize those calories and activate fat-burning potential. Or, their metabolisms may be so slow because of chronic stress that they cannot burn the calories effectively. Either way, you've got a fat-storing crisis.

Living life in the fast lane (and often, the fast-food lane) means that food choices are often based on convenience instead of nutrition. That not only means a junk-food diet, but a junk diet: lots of calories, lots of fat, lots of sodium, lots of sugar—all promising energy on the run. But the energy runs out and ends up slowing down, not speeding up, our metabolism.

The classic junk diet is notoriously low in the nutrients that provide for consistent, long-lasting energy. We are more likely to eat fries than baked potatoes, ketchup than tomatoes, and drink orange soda instead of orange juice. So most of us are deficient in the vitamins and minerals that would keep our metabolism working in high gear.

But we can choose to eat well and eat often. To preserve muscle mass and burn fat while losing weight, your best bet is to eat balanced meals and snacks of whole carbohydrates and low-fat protein, evenly distributed throughout the day. This, in combination with eating an adequate amount of calories, is the most important step you can take to unleash your body's natural ability to lose weight.

To activate your metabolism and get your body working for you, you need to eat The Smart Weigh. That means you need to: 1. eat early, 2. eat often, 3. eat balanced, 4. eat lean, and 5. eat bright. (You can read more about strategic eating in Chapter 3.)

Fanning the Fire's Flame

Eating strategically is one of the best ways to increase your metabolism, and exercise is a close second. Yet, research shows that most people with weight problems not only eat too much, too late, but exercise too little. If you're serious about losing weight and keeping it off, you must eat right and exercise. You can't do one or the other. Controlling your intake of food is not an alternative to exercise, nor is exercise an alternative to healthy eating.

Not only does exercise help you to burn the calories you take in better, it also serves to build muscle mass. And that's another weight-control secret: To rev up your metabolism and burn fat, use—don't lose—your muscle. Building new muscle through strength training is one of the best ways to reverse the metabolic slowdown of midlife and stressful living. The more lean muscle mass you can preserve, the bigger "engine" you'll have in which to burn calories.

Now, does what you've always heard about the importance of exercise make more sense? You can boost your metabolism, lose body fat, and gain muscle mass by doing some type of aerobic activity for thirty to sixty minutes at least four times a week. No time? Break up your workouts into shorter bouts throughout the day. Reports show that squeezing in even ten-minute spurts of activity throughout the day yields results. Add in a workout with free weights, exercise bands, or a Nautilus machine twice a week, or take advantage of the humdrum tasks that have to be done anyway by doing them with vigor. Haul the garbage cans to the curb yourself and rejoice when you carry that laundry basket up and down the stairs! Even though regularly scheduled aerobic exercise is best for losing fat, any extra movement boosts the metabolism and burns calories better. Start parking at the far end of the lot, or make several trips up and down the stairs instead of using the elevator. Even foregoing such automated gadgets as remote controls and garage door openers can make a metabolic difference. (Read more about the benefits of movement in Chapter 4.)

Taking Care of Yourself

You might be wondering, "Where am I going to get the energy to do all this extra moving and working out? I can barely keep my pace as it is!" You're not alone. Not only are many of us living in metabolic lockdown as a result of our lifestyle choices, we're living in an energy crisis as well. The very things that result in a slowed metabolism produce the energy deficit, too. One of these factors is sleep deprivation. (You'll read more about the power of restful sleep in Chapter 6.)

Sleep is the repair shop of the body; without it we cannot be healthy or even happy. Sleep deprivation actually becomes a profound stress to your body, contributing to fat cell lockdown. Research shows that missing just one night of restful sleep can cause a surge of stress hormones to circulate through your body, weakening your immune system and causing a metabolic slowdown. Conversely, replenishing sleep and timeouts can equip the body for stress release. It's how we were created.

Breathing is another normal body action that can either release stress or actually cause it. You can't help breathing, but you can help yourself breathe better. Taking deep, slow, oxygenating breaths is one of the simplest things you can do to relieve stress, activate your metabolism, and keep control of yourself in any situation.

Yet in times of stress, we tend to breathe in a panicked way—rapid, shallow, or deep, heaving breaths, each breath robbing the bloodstream of the right amount of oxygen to take to the cells to fan the metabolic fire. You can think of this kind of stress breathing as suffocating your blood cells—which signals the release of even more stress hormones. The more stressed and tense you are, the higher your brain's demand for oxygen, yet the shallow breathing that accompanies stress decreases the oxygen intake and transfer. It's a vicious cycle that takes your breath away! The good news is that you can learn how to breathe in a relaxed way that immediately defuses the stress response. (Read more about the healing benefits of focused breathing in Chapter 5.)

Drinking adequate amounts of water is another critical element for activating your metabolism and total body health. Because your body is composed primarily of water, every cell in your body relies on this "one-of-a-kind" beverage to dilute biochemicals, vitamins, and minerals to just the right concentrations so they can be used in energy metabolism. The body also depends on water to keep blood at the proper fluid concentration to transport these nutrients and other substances effectively from one part to another. Blood volume actually decreases and "thickens" when you are dehydrated, meaning that the heart has to work harder to supply your cells with needed oxygen. And remember, oxygenated blood is essential for an activated metabolism—to fan the flame for fat burning. A slow-burning metabolism is a symptom of dehydration.

By now you're getting the picture: activating your metabolism is really just a matter of moving into better self-care. That means treating yourself well by eating right, drinking enough water, exercising and strengthening your body, breathing deeply, and getting rest. The opposite behavior—a lack of self-care—is the recipe for fat storage.

2. Regulate Your Blood Sugars

Our blood sugar level is one of the more powerful influences on our well-being, our ability to lose weight, and our appetite. From a chemical perspective, regulating our blood sugar level is the most effective way to release our fat-burning capacity.

When our blood sugars are up and even, but not too high, we are brimming with energy and vitality and our appetite is in control. When the levels are bouncing widely and wildly, our energy, mood, memory, clarity of thought, and overall performance are likely to rise and fall along with them.

Blood sugar levels normally crest and fall every three to four hours, and even more often and intensely when your body is stuck in the stress response. As sugars fall, so will your sense of well-being, energy level, concentration, and ability to handle stress. Your body will need about half an hour to convert what you eat to energy, so waiting to eat until you're cranky and starving doesn't help immediately. If you've starved all day, the drop in sugars will be a "free fall," leaving you weak, sleepy, dizzy, and hungry. There's one thing that doesn't fall with blood sugars, and that's your appetite. As the blood sugars crash, the body sends a chemical signal to the brain's appetite control center, demanding to be fed. And your cells are screaming for a quick energy source—not broccoli or cauliflower, but chocolate chips or Reese's Peanut Butter Cups!

Too much sugar and refined carbohydrates is a drain on anyone's energy metabolism, and a serious one for people with sensitive blood sugar responses. Once a person who is sensitive to the rises and falls in blood sugar has eaten, his or her blood sugar rises quickly—very quickly if the person has consumed a refined carbohydrate with a high glycemic index (one that is "fast-released" into the bloodstream as glucose). And that's the problem: what comes up quickly will quickly come down. These quick bursts of energy can ultimately cause fatigue and stimulate appetite by creating a drop in blood sugar due to surges in the hormone insulin, which accelerates the conversion of calories into fat. Insulin levels rise in response to the higher blood glucose level that moves the sugar into the cell to be processed. The insulin does so by opening muscle cell doors wide to usher in the glucose that is to be burned for energy. But if you've consumed more calories than you can use at that time for energy, the insulin ushers the calories into the fat cells to be stored as fat. If you're also overloading on fat, those fat cell doors swing open wider still.

Everyone responds poorly to a high glucose load, but some respond worse than others. To estimate how blood sugar will be affected by eating, the glycemic potential of food has been established to show whether a food will raise blood sugar levels dramatically and quickly (fast release), moderately (quick release), or just a little (slow release). The glycemic rating of pure sugar is set at 100, and every other food is ranked on a scale from 0 to 100, based on its effect on blood sugars. Carbohydrates that break down quickly during digestion have the highest glycemic values—the level of glucose in the blood increases rapidly when these foods are eaten. On the other hand, carbohydrates that break down slowly, releasing glucose gradually into the bloodstream, have low glycemic ratings. The fast-releasing carbohydrates will be ranked with a glycemic index of more than 70, quick-release carbs rank between 55 and 70, and slow-release carbohydrates are given a rating below 55. The higher the number, the faster the blood sugars rise.

When the blood sugar rise is fast, the insulin released into the bloodstream is abundant. The high insulin level will outlast the sugar burst, taking more and more sugar into the cells and dramatically dropping the blood sugar levels to a less than desirable level. The result is that the person soon feels spacey, unable to concentrate, weak, sleepy, anxious, sweaty, or dizzy. The quick drop in blood sugar will also trigger a craving for more carbohydrates, the essence of what is termed sugar or carbohydrate "addiction." In addition, the higher levels of circulating insulin stimulate the storage of fat in the cells and inhibit the burning of fat as energy. This is why eating evenly and wisely will keep blood sugar and insulin levels in check and enable the body to burn fat and release optimal energy.

FOODS LOW ON THE GLYCEMIC INDEX

Some foods produce a lower glycemic response than others—meaning that they result in a lower insulin surge—and are considered smart choices for day-by-day eating, especially for those seeking stable blood sugars and lower insulin levels. I consider those foods with a glycemic index ranking under 55 to be the better choices.

BETTER CHOICE GRAINS
Oats
Barley
Buckwheat
Uncle Sam's Cereal
Kellogg's Bran Buds with psyllium
Bulgur
Long grain brown or basmati rice
Tortilla
Whole wheat or artichoke pasta
100 percent stoneground whole
    wheat bread
Whole grain pumpernickel bread
Whole wheat sourdough bread

BETTER CHOICE LEGUMES
Chick peas
Kidney beans
Lentils
Navy beans
Soybeans *(the best!)*
Peanuts

BETTER CHOICE VEGETABLES
Carrots
Corn
Green peas
Lima beans
Sweet potatoes
Yams

BETTER CHOICE FRUITS
Apples
Apricots, dried
Small banana
Cherries
Grapefruit
Grapes
Kiwis
Mangos
Oranges
Peaches
Pears
Plums
Tomatoes

The information regarding the glycemic response of food and the body's resulting chemical response is not just a theory or based on preliminary results of research. It is fact, the documented results of many studies that have been published in medical and scientific journals around the world. Most of the popular diet plans and books written in the past decade have addressed the hormonal response to food and attempted to solve it in different ways, but the attempts are almost always knee-jerk reactions causing pendulum swings. Cutting out all carbohydrates is not the answer, because all carbohydrates are not the problem. It's the unbalanced diet that's the problem: refined carbohydrates are being eaten to excess, and the excess calories are being stored as fat.

The key to long-term weight loss and maintenance is to get plenty of carbohydrates—but make them whole and don't overload. Their intake needs to be balanced with low-fat proteins. Eating the right proteins increases your level of glucagon, another hormone that works to lower your insulin level. If you eat lunches that are high in refined carbohydrates but low in protein, you will throw off the glucagon-insulin balance and may find yourself feeling tired and craving sweets in the afternoon. It's a normal physical reaction. So keep your metabolism, fat-burning capacity, energy, and concentration up, and appetite and cravings down, throughout your day by eating small amounts more often.

3. Take Charge of Your Appetite

Many people go wrong not in what they eat, but in how much they eat. Even if they are eating food that is good for them, they often eat too much of it. Calories do count, so learning how to say "enough"—before you've eaten way too much—is vital.

Although this advice may seem contradictory at first, the way to tame your appetite and stop overeating is to start eating. It's a fact: wise eating all through the day keeps ravenous appetite away. Enjoying food, not shunning it, is the answer. I know that can strike fear in the heart of any overeater who believes that once he or she begins to eat, there is no stopping. And who has time to eat so often anyway?

American society has become so focused on avoiding and getting rid of fat that we've lost the positive and pleasurable aspects of eating. We've settled for foods that are convenient yet incapable of providing the full sensory experience. And that leads to one thing: overeating. When you've pushed your body through the day on fumes and eat steamed vegetables and plain broiled chicken night after night, pizza and Haagen-Dazs can sound really good—and a lot of it sounds better! Starvation and sensory deprivation are sure routes to a binge.

Managing Cravings

Most of us have experienced a strong, nearly uncontrollable urge for a certain type of food. And while we've struggled to keep away from the

LIQUID SNACKS?

Don't make the mistake of slugging down soda to keep from snacking on candy or chips, thinking that at least it's fat free. (The average American downs fifty-three gallons of soda a year: 79,146 empty calories!)

In a recent study at Purdue University, subjects were fed extra calories in the form of solid food every day for a month. Their total daily calorie intake—and their weight—remained stable. They made up for the snack calories by cutting back elsewhere in their diets.

During a different month, they were given the same number of extra calories, but this time in a liquid form. Their total calorie intake went up, and they put on pounds. The reason, in theory, is that liquids pass through the digestive tract too quickly to trigger a feeling of satiety, so the "take in more" signal persists.

Other studies have shown that even people who drink diet sodas eat more calories. Of course, diet soda itself has no calories, but the sweet taste can trigger an insulin release that signals you to eat more—which is one of the many reasons that diet sodas have not produced a fit and trim world.

Some solid advice: choose snacks you can chew.

refrigerator, we may have wondered why we long so intensely for a particular taste. Why do we have cravings? Are they emotional or physical?

Most people don't sell their soul for a stalk of celery. They are driven toward sugar and salt (inborn preferences for infants to drink breast milk) and fat (inborn preferences for children to sustain growth). The problem is that even though children outgrow their biological needs, their tastes persist because of the foods that are cultural and family favorites. They develop passions for peanut butter and jelly, macaroni and cheese, cheeseburgers, and milkshakes. For the more sophisticated palates of adults, it's Rocky Road ice cream, fettuccine alfredo, nachos, and creamy chocolate mousse.

Diet deficiencies fuel the cravings. As you've read, fluctuating blood sugars—enhanced by unbalanced hormones and stress chemicals—stimulate the driving desire for sweets; fluid imbalances drive the desire for salty foods; a sustained inadequate intake of calories (lack of supply to meet demands) fuels the desire for fats. This is the physical side of the craving, driving us in a general direction.

Our emotions help determine the exact food we decide on. The body sends out the "I NEED" signal, the emotions send out the "I WANT" signal, and both send us directly to the comfort food of choice, particularly when comfort is being called for. Our culture's battle cry is "relief is just a swallow away," and for many of us that spells food. The refrigerator light becomes the light of our life.

The 10 Commandments of Satisfied Eating

It takes time to recognize the emotional issues behind the "I WANT" signal, but you can take charge of the physical side of your appetite this very day by learning to recognize true hunger. If you've been eating too much, too frequently, or too infrequently, it will take some time and adjustments to learn—and obey—your true hunger signals. Everyone is different; your task is to watch for your own unique hunger and satisfaction clues.

Hunger is not always about stomach sensations; it's more often about energy drops, weakness, fatigue, bad concentration, an empty feeling, crankiness, even cold hands and feet. Satiation has occurred when there is an absence of hunger or fullness, a level of physical energy, loss of interest in food, and interest in other things. You are more than likely overfull (or as my teen-age daughter calls it, "at capacity") when you are feeling bloated, lethargic, and short of breath. Your healthy goal is to eat to your level of satiation. Eat balanced and choose wisely, but stop when you are satisfied.

When you're eating right things at the right time, your meals and snacks will satisfy you much more easily. If you find you are feeling hungry between regularly scheduled meals and snacks, wait ten minutes and see if you still are. After ten minutes, ask yourself if there is something going on emotionally—or if you are just bored or stressed. If you're truly hungry, have your power snack at that time, even if you need to add another to that day.

You don't have to rely on iron-willed discipline to control your food intake. By following an eating plan that meets the physical needs of your body, you will be in control. Follow these ten tips to stay full—and satisfied:

1. Keep a log on the fire all day. The eat-right prescription of eating early and often, balanced and lean, with lots of brightly colored fruits and vegetables will fill you with satisfying protein, appetite-curbing fiber, and energy-boosting carbohydrates. And mini-meals or power snacks every couple of hours will keep your metabolism in high gear and your appetite in control. Don't be a rabbit—salad alone won't satisfy you. Eat a well-balanced diet with plenty of fiber.

2. Eat fruit before every meal. These satisfying tidbits can curb your appetite and slow down your eating. Listen to your body and focus on fueling *it* rather than feeding your emotional needs. Remember, it takes most people about twenty minutes to feel full. We often eat too much in three to five minutes, and are left still looking for more. The simple carbohydrates in your fruit appetizer will have reached your bloodstream by then, helping you to reach satisfaction without looking for something sweet.

3. Pay attention to your food. Inhaling a sandwich at your desk or in your car can set you up for overeating—it fills you up, but doesn't satisfy you. We often turn to richly flavored candy bars or fat-filled chips to satisfy the flavor needs we didn't get during our meal. Instead, take the time to focus on what you're eating and savor every bite. And make it great! Forego bland and tasteless, albeit quick and easy, meals. Go for flavor and pizzazz!

4. Have a seat. Rushing through a meal can leave you feeling deprived even when your body's signaling that you're full. Savor your food, and avoid distractions like watching TV, which encourages mindless eating. Try to dine at the dinner table only. If you always eat in front of the TV, then every time you nestle in with the remote control, it's a cue to eat. Instead, designate an eating spot for all meals and snacks.

5. Drink water, drink water, drink water. And a lot of it! Don't mistake dehydration for hunger. If you yearn for salty foods, a big craving catalyst is probably your lack of proper fluids, which depletes your body's sodium supply. If you're craving chips, try a tall glass of water first! And have a tall glass of water before and after each meal.

6. Wait out cravings. Think before you bite. Creating rituals—like the old standby of waiting ten minutes before giving in to a craving—can stop you from eating when you aren't really hungry. Ask before you reach: Are you bored, tired, angry, stressed, or lonely? If so, you won't find the answer in food. If you find that your emotions are fueling your cravings, choose a healthier alternative than overeating. Sure, you can eat a bag of Oreos when you're angry or frustrated, but a five-minute walk will work, too. And you'll feel better, not bloated.

If the craving seems stronger than you are, try to make the most of it. If you crave ice cream, choose sorbet and yogurt and top it with fresh fruit. If you crave chips, get the baked version and have them with a fat-free bean dip or top them with melted low-fat cheese. Give yourself a treat, not a trick.

7. **Talk to yourself.** At heart, we all crave continuity. So when you try to alter long-standing eating habits, inner voices will pipe up to protest the change. Try to remember specifically why you want to change your eating habits (e.g., "I'll have more energy when I lose weight").

8. **Exercise.** Regular exercise keeps you energized and may even suppress your appetite for several hours. Exercise boosts your brain's production of serotonin, a feel-good brain chemical that increases concentration and energy while reducing carbohydrate cravings.

9. **Put a mirror on the fridge.** It may sound strange, but researchers found that people who ate at a table with a large mirror on it were more likely to choose reduced-fat or fat-free products than those higher in fat or calories. That doesn't mean that you need to hang a mirror by the dining room table. A small mirror on your refrigerator or inside the pantry door may get the message across. Keeping a food diary can also serve as a sort of mirror for your eating patterns, helping you get a grip on your eating reality.

10. **Be patient.** Very, very patient! Forget quick diet fixes—it can take three to six months to replace bad habits with healthy ones. Answering the call of an appetite that's run wild is a physical as well as habitual pattern; it takes time to learn how to turn down your personal appetite thermostat, and time to learn how to "just say no" to urges that aren't physical at all. The quickest way to become discouraged is to expect quick success. So give yourself plenty of time to change. This will increase the odds that you'll stay motivated for the long run.

Welcome to The Smart Weigh

The Smart Weigh plan is not a magic formula. It is a nondieting solution to weight management that works to unleash your body's natural healing and weight-loss mechanism. It is based on timeless truths that show you how the body was designed to work and how you can choose food and water, exercise, air, rest, and self-care to work for you, not against you. It enables you to operate from a point of strength physically—and sets the stage for you to meet the deeper needs of your soul.

I won't give you a specific diet to follow because sooner or later you have to go off it—you know that. But I do ask you to do this: throw out your diet books, and just say no to the next "diet answer" that comes to you via your friends, family, or group. Make the decision, today, to turn from the dieting path, and take a small step on the road to looking and feeling better. Refuse to sacrifice your health and your energy at the altar of improper weight loss.

Embrace these simple truths: live The Smart Weigh.

The Smart Weigh in Action

S: Strategic Eating
M: Movement
A: Air and Water
R: Rest
T: Treat Yourself Well

Is The Smart Weigh easy? Quite honestly, because this lifestyle and eating plan represents the ultimate in health and nutrition, you'll probably find The Smart Weigh plan a challenge at first, as you adopt some new, powerfully healthy habits. But the results will be worth it. Studies show that each improvement in lifestyle will not only help your weight loss, but will also lower your risk of heart attack, high blood pressure, stroke, cancer, diabetes, osteoporosis, cataracts, asthma, diverticulosis, depression, and even PMS.

Many of the specific steps outlined in The Smart Weigh program will help you change your attitude or lifestyle, which in turn will help crack the code of the fat cell. You have to start somewhere—and The Smart Weigh is that place.

CHAPTER 2

JUMP-START
YOUR LIFE,
THE SMART WEIGH

THERE'S A GOOD REASON why most people fail at sustaining a new way of living: they don't plan to fail, but fail to plan. The best way to reach long-term goals is with short-term steps. But most people try to make changes without understanding that changing behavior is a process, not a once-a-year New Year's resolution.

And often, they don't really understand *what* behaviors they're trying to change. That's absolutely critical. If your current diet is loaded with sugar or caffeine, for example, you need to know that it won't be easy at first to change how you eat.

So the very first step on the path to living The Smart Weigh is an honest assessment of where you are *today*. You can't set a course for where you want to go if you don't know where you are. And there's only one way to do that: write it down. For one week, keep a diary of everything you eat and drink, the time that you eat, how you are feeling, and any exercise you may do.

Do this now, before you start implementing any of the changes in this book. As you keep track of how you are living each day, look for the areas that may be contributing to your metabolism slow-down and fat cell lockdown. What patterns do you see with your eating, your exercise, your moods, and your feelings? Do you snack on candy bars and sodas for an instant energy boost? And do you find yourself feeling fatigued and in need of another boost a few hours later? If you do, there's a very good reason.

Breaking the Grip of Sugar and Caffeine

One of the biggest blunders we make in eating isn't about eating at all. It's about depending on food for a chemical brain boost to get us through the rough times when energy is low and we're being dealt some bad cards. The two prime examples of substances we give too much power to are sugar and caffeine. Let's take a look at breaking their grip.

Know that withdrawal is real. If you are sugar sensitive and caffeine-dependent, you are apt to experience physical symptoms of drug deprivation. You may feel shaky, nauseous, fatigued, or edgy, or experience headaches or diarrhea.

As you embark on any healthy lifestyle change—especially one as chemically impacting as pulling back from a high intake of sugar or caffeine—your body needs time to adjust physiologically and emotionally. You can expect the following changes.

On Days 1 and 2, you may feel slightly sluggish, irritable, and dissatisfied with your eating. Day 3 will be one of your most difficult days, as your body begins to feel the chemical change. It may seem that every cell in your body is crying out for food, particularly something sweet. But the urge for sweets is not impossible to overcome. If you make it through the third day without overeating or homicide, it gets better. At the end of this chapter, I'll offer a three-day meal plan to help you jump-start your new life, The Smart Weigh.

I know these symptoms may sound more like withdrawal from hard drugs than from simply allowing your body to adjust to a wonderfully healthy way of eating. But let's face reality: Putting in healthy foods means leaving out the unhealthy, and that means a chemical change—a withdrawal of sorts. If you recognize that the chemical changes are necessary, but temporary, it will be easier for you to break through to a lifetime of good eating. Again, that's why it's necessary to keep a one-week diary first, so you'll know whether sugar or caffeine withdrawal is likely to be a problem for you.

Know when you're vulnerable. Identify—and avoid—resolve-breakers like fatigue, hunger, anger, or loneliness. If you need something when you're tired, to "get through," break for a nap—even if it is more difficult—rather than reaching for the cookies. If you have spent a lifetime pushing down anger with food, then it's time to switch to the more difficult but healthier choice: Write away your anger in a journal or discuss its cause with someone.

Know that it will get easier. Although we are born with a natural preference toward foods with a sweet taste, these preferences have been overdeveloped and fueled by a lifetime of high sugar intake and erratic eating patterns. As you cut back, over time, your cravings diminish and your taste buds regain their ability to pick up the sweetness in a carrot or piece of fruit.

"Power snack" throughout the day. I'll say this over and over throughout this book: Eating every two to three hours throughout the day keeps your energy okay and a ravenous appetite away. Go for energy-boosting combos like fresh fruit or a box of raisins with low-fat cheese or yogurt, a half sandwich, or a trail mix of dry-roasted peanuts and sunflower seeds mixed with dried fruit. Keep power snacks like these available wherever you are—they will serve as a lift to your body and prevent the drowsiness and sweet cravings that often follow meals.

Are You a Java Junkie?

Caffeine is among the world's most widely used and addictive drugs. It keeps you alert by blocking one of the brain's natural sedatives, a neurotransmitter called adenosine. It stimulates the central nervous system, increases your pulse rate and heartbeat, and can even give quite a boost to your mood. A single cup of coffee can seem to work energy miracles when needed—even helping athletes to push a little farther. All in all, it's powerful stuff.

But there is a downside to caffeine: too much causes a surge of adrenaline. And when the spurt is over, power levels plummet and stress hormones are produced. Even small amounts of caffeine may cause side effects, including restlessness and disturbed sleep, heart palpitations, stomach irritation, fibrocystic breast disease, and diarrhea. It can promote irritability, anxiety, and mood disturbances. Caffeine can also aggravate premenstrual syndrome and mood swings in women. And studies have shown that the stress hormones circulate, elevating blood pressure, up to eight hours after the last caffeine hit. And those stress hormones play a key role in fat cell lockdown.

The stimulant effect is thought to kick in with consumption of 150 to 250 mg of caffeine—the amount in one mug of brewed coffee or three glasses of iced tea. And because caffeine is also found in soda (regular and diet), chocolate, and even decongestant cold pills, it adds up quickly. The levels soar when you get java from a gourmet coffee shop. New analysis shows that these specialty brews can contain two to three times the caffeine found in a cup made from your typical supermarket brands. These specialty coffees are stronger because more grounds are used to give the brew its rich flavor and the beans are often roasted, making the coffee even more potent. In fact, one large cup of specialty coffee packs a walloping 280 mg of caffeine, and some have been found to contain 550 mg. It's at these higher levels of intake, about 600 mg, that you can get too energized and start to feel the java jitters: frazzled nerves, the shakes, insomnia, and ultimately, fatigue.

Do you need to cut out caffeine altogether? Not necessarily. Despite its drawbacks, it's definitely an energy boost. My concern is when caffeine becomes your very best friend. I do encourage you to cut back slowly to a ceiling of 250 mg. And if, after cutting back to this amount, you still experience any of the above-mentioned effects, I would suggest withdrawing altogether. You'll also get more of an energy boost from the caffeine you do consume if you cut back on your intake.

Pain is the word that best characterizes cutting back on caffeine consumption, and that is why you must do so gradually. Again, caffeine is a powerfully addictive drug that will bring withdrawal symptoms as you give it up. Many people experience zombie-like fatigue, irritability, lethargy, and headaches from going "cold turkey," and the symptoms may last up to five days. They expect to feel better by nobly giving up espresso, but end up feeling horrible instead. Then they drag back to caffeine saying this "healthy thing" just didn't work for them.

Cut back slowly over the course of a week to ten days. Start by cutting back to a safer level of two cups of coffee or three cups of tea. Gradually cut back, a quarter of a cup at a time, until you are down to none. Or substitute a decaffeinated product for the real thing in the same reducing amounts. Withdrawal will be less painful if you follow The Smart Weigh meal plan. Eating small, balanced meals throughout the day will stabilize your body chemistries and reduce your reliance on caffeine for energy. And, if you focus on drinking more water than you have in the past, you won't have room for the other beverages. In addition, try to get outdoor exercise every day to get a boost of feel-good endorphins.

Three Days

In the chapters that follow, I'll discuss in detail the principles of The Smart Weigh that will help you understand why you feel the way you do. And I'll provide a seven-week plan to guide you on your personal quest to shed unwanted pounds, gain energy, feel better, and recapture the joy of living.

But I know how hard it is to look seven days down the road, much less seven weeks. So for now, I just want you to give me three days. Three days that can change your life. Consider this a sneak preview, if you will. As I said, you'll find the complete seven-week plan in Chapter 8. But for now, read over the first three days below. This shows you in detail how to get started, how to begin the process of changing behaviors it may have taken you years to develop. Before you set a start date for your new life, before you commit to living The Smart Weigh, you must be willing to commit to three days. You won't regret it. The rewards will last a lifetime.

The Smart Weigh Jump-start Plan

Day One

The moment you are vertical: Drink 8 ounces of warm water with lemon, then a 6-ounce glass of white grape juice.

Breakfast (within ½ hour of rising): Scrambled Egg Burrito (page 170) OR 1 slice whole-grain toast topped with 2 ounces of melted, low-fat cheese, and 1 small apple or pear.

Midmorning Snack (2½ hours later): 1 small banana with 2 ounces of low-fat cheese or soy cheese.

Lunch (2½ hours later): 1 sliced orange as an appetizer, 1 turkey tortilla roll (3 ounces of turkey rolled into 1 whole-wheat, fat-free tortilla, spread with Dijon mustard, with shredded lettuce and tomato), plus cut-up raw veggies to munch on.

Midafternoon Snack (2½ hours later): ¼ cup Trail Mix (1 Tbs. dry-roasted peanuts or soy nuts, 1 Tbs. sunflower or pumpkin seeds, 2 Tbs. raisins).

Dinner (2½ hours later): 1 cup melon as an appetizer. Try Herb-Crusted Orange Roughy on page 176 OR 2-3 ounces of grilled fish, 1 small baked sweet potato topped with cinnamon, 1 cup steamed broccoli, green salad drizzled with low-fat balsamic dressing.

Bedtime Snack (½ hour before bedtime): ½ cup whole-grain cereal and ½ cup skim or soy milk.

Day Two

Breakfast (within ½ hour of arising): Power shake (page 169)

Midmorning Snack (2½ hours later): 5 whole-grain crackers with 2 ounces of low-fat cheese or soy cheese.

Lunch (2½ hours later): ¼ cantaloupe as an appetizer, 1 whole wheat pita pocket packed with romaine, tomato and ¾ cup tuna salad (made with water-packed solid white tuna, with 1 Tbs. light mayonnaise, Dijon mustard, chopped red peppers, and spices to taste), raw vegetables to munch on.

Midafternoon Snack (2½ hours later): 3 cups microwave light popcorn sprinkled with 2 Tbs. Parmesan cheese.

Dinner (2½ hours later): 8-ounce glass of V-8 or tomato juice as an appetizer. Try Chicken Laurent on page 179 OR 2-3 ounces of grilled chicken, ½ cup steamed brown rice, 1 cup steamed asparagus or spinach, green salad drizzled with low-fat balsamic dressing.

Bedtime Snack (½ hour before bedtime): ½ cup whole-grain cereal and ½ cup skim or soy milk.

Day Three

The moment you are vertical: Drink 8 ounces of warm water with lemon, then a 6-ounce glass of white grape juice.

Breakfast (within ½ hour of arising): Hot Apple Cinnamon Oatmeal (page 173).

Midmorning Snack (2½ hours later): 8 ounces Stonyfield Farms Yogurt (or 8 ounces plain yogurt mixed with 1 Tbs. all-fruit jam)

Lunch (2½ hours later): ¾ cup berries as an appetizer
Large Romaine salad with sliced tomato topped with 3 ounces grilled chicken, low-fat balsamic vinegar or salsa for dressing, 5 whole grain crackers or 1 ounce baked tortilla chips.

Midafternoon Snack: 1 turkey tortilla roll (1 ounces of turkey rolled into 1 whole-wheat, fat-free tortilla, spread with Dijon mustard, with shredded lettuce and tomato).

Dinner: Try Poached Salmon over Black Bean Salad (page 181) or 8 large steamed or grilled shrimp, 1 ear of cooked corn, 1 cup spinach. Try Apple Walnut Salad (page 182) or 1 sliced apple and a green salad.

Bedtime Snack (½ hour before bedtime): ½ cup whole-grain cereal and ½ cup skim or soy milk.

Now that you're three days strong, read on to discover why you're feeling so much better and why The Smart Weigh is your answer for losing weight without losing your soul.

CHAPTER 3

STRATEGIC EATING

S
M
A
R
T

WHAT IF WE STOPPED TRYING not to eat, or not to cheat, and started planning how best to charge up our internal motor? Then we'd be eating The Smart Weigh—and feel great all day, relax and play all evening, and rise to almost any occasion, with activated metabolisms and bodies that are working for us and with us.

Eating smart isn't about what you shouldn't be eating; it's not about how bad potato chips or ice cream or red meat may be for you. Instead, it's about the foods and lifestyle choices that power you with high-octane energy fuel. The food you eat shapes the optimal performance and effectiveness of all your body mechanisms and allows your metabolism to burn in high gear. Releasing your body's natural ability to lose weight requires a nutrition plan that goes far beyond traditional or fad dieting.

It was only a decade ago that the world of nutrition began to go beyond dieting for weight loss alone and to focus instead on living life well each day while preventing the diseases of tomorrow.

Most of us underestimate the effect of our eating on how we feel. We don't connect morning sluggishness or afternoon sleepiness to when and what we eat. We know that food is our body's fuel, but most of us resist an even flow. As our schedules get full, it's easy for a consistent eating routine to go awry. Eating falls into an erratic, catch-as-catch-can affair that can't supply our body's needs. It seems as if we can't afford the time to eat well, yet the truth is that we can't afford not to. Wisely chosen food is a powerful tool to right the wrong of stress, and remove the logjam to your metabolism that it causes. Paying attention to how you eat is a small-time investment with a tremendous return.

Right now, changing your eating patterns may seem like just another duty, maybe even another diet. But you will find that choosing to eat the right foods at the right time is choosing freedom. Making wise choices and exercising self-control frees you to be the real you—free from compulsive dieting, overeating, or self-abusive living. Thousands of people have done it—and you can, too!

Edible Energy

When it comes to nutrition, calories take a lot of abuse. Most Americans, particularly women, want to cut them, burn them, and otherwise get rid of them. But a certain number of calories are essential. They provide the fuel our bodies need in order to function. The truth about food is simple: Food is just tasty units of energy. It takes food to make energy and to activate the metabolism.

The food we eat gets converted to glucose, which is the brain and lungs' only energy source and the most efficient and common form for the rest of the body. A single molecule of glucose can trigger the production of nearly thirty-eight molecules of ATP, the energy molecule that fuels the body's cells. Without ATP, the cells go on a hunger strike and muscles stiffen, refusing to function efficiently. Our moment-by-moment personal energy is, at the most basic level,

all about how much ATP our body is producing. Food—and calories—give us the power to breathe, think, move, crack a joke, make
love. Taken in appropriate amounts at the proper times, they are a
very good thing.

Three components in foods provide calories: carbohydrates, proteins, and fats. Per gram (about the weight of a paper clip), each
component provides the following number of calories:

Carbohydrates: 4 calories per gram
Protein: 4 calories per gram
Fat: 9 calories per gram

Alcohol also provides calories—7 calories per gram—but no nutritive value. Generally speaking, all calories—whether from carbohydrates, proteins, or fats—supply the same amount of energy. But each
makes unique contributions to bodily function and health. Foods
high in carbohydrates (including breads and starches) are mostly used
for energy. The fiber that is found in many high-carbohydrate foods
also helps regulate bowel function and protects against heart disease
and certain types of cancer. Carbohydrates should make up about 55
to 60 percent of your total daily calories.

Protein (including meats, legumes, and soybean products) may
also be used for energy. But the body uses protein in more vital
ways—to make and maintain body tissue such as muscles and
organs. In addition, protein is a key component of enzymes, hormones, and many body fluids. When there are enough calories from
other sources, the body uses protein for these essential purposes
rather than for fuel. Only about 15 to 20 percent of your daily calories should come from protein.

Fat provides the most concentrated source of energy. Even a little fat can provide a lot of calories. In excess, fat can increase the
risk of cardiovascular disease and some cancers. Fat comes in two
forms: saturated and unsaturated. No more than 30 percent of
your daily calories should come from fat, and—ideally—no more

HOW TO REACH YOUR TARGET WEIGHT

To calculate if you are getting enough fuel, use this formula: multiply your current weight by 16 if you're active, by 12 if you exercise by lifting the remote control. This gives you the approximate number of calories you typically burn in a day—and the amount that will give optimal energy and the amount needed to maintain your current weight. An active 125-pound woman burns roughly 2,000 calories, a sedentary one will need only 1,750. An active 175-pound man needs 2,800 calories, a sedentary one will need only 2,100. To gain one pound per week, 500 calories should be added daily; to lose one pound per week, 500 calories should be cut daily—never to less than 1,500 calories for a female or 1,800 calories for a male.

Eating less than 1,500 calories per day can slow down your metabolic rate by 30 percent and leave you without key energy-releasing nutrients. Your memory, concentration, and judgment can all be impaired. Since weight loss means cutting back on those valuable energy-giving calories, it requires upping the ante of quality and timing of eating. To make up the difference, the goal is to become more active and better burn the calories consumed.

than 20 to 25 percent.

Caloric needs vary considerably from one individual to another. A small, elderly, sedentary woman requires fewer calories than a large, young, physically active man. The number of calories you need depends on your age, height, weight, gender, and activity level. But remember, it's not just the energy consumed that counts, it's the energy burned. As we've discussed, our stressful, frenzied, and often sedentary lifestyles have slowed our metabolic rate to a snail's pace, resulting in fats being stored rather than burned for energy.

We need to activate our metabolism with The Smart Weigh eat-right prescription: small meals of high-energy, whole-grain carbohydrates, and power-building, low-fat proteins complemented by brightly colored fruits and vegetables, at least every three hours, with LOTS of water.

To reach your target weight, first figure out how many calories to cut to hit your goal. One pound of fat equals approximately 3,500 calories. Multiply 3,500 by the number of pounds you want to shed. To lose five pounds you'd need to burn about 17,500 calories. If you cut 500 calories daily below what you need for maintenance, you could lose the weight in about five weeks.

An easier approach is to split the equation. By shaving calories from your food intake and simultaneously becoming more active, you can minimize the struggle and maximize the results—reaching your goal sooner. The Smart Weigh plan uses the dynamic duo: reducing calories by 250 to 750 per day and burning an additional 250 calories with added exercise.

To Lose	You Need to Use	Exercising Only Time to Goal Weight	Exercising & Eating Well Time to Goal Weight
5 pounds	17,500 calories	6 weeks	4 weeks
10 pounds	35,000 calories	12 weeks	8 weeks
20 pounds	70,000 calories	24 weeks	16 weeks

Eat Early

Although it may not seem like news, breakfast is still the most important meal of your day: Don't leave home without it! Breakfast begins your day by stabilizing body chemistries and starting your metabolism in high gear. View eating breakfast as a primary metabolic booster. After a night's sleep, it takes 250 to 350 calories to get your metabolism percolating again.

If you choose not to eat breakfast, your body turns to internal sources for energy, burning muscle mass (not fat) for fuel. The metabolism slows down another notch, conserving itself in this disabled, starved state. Continuing to starve your body will leave it dragging through the day, unable to work efficiently and more ready to store whatever food is eaten. If you consume most of your calories in the evening, much of the nutrients you eat will be wasted and the energy stored as fat. All that food can't possibly be used up because your body isn't burning energy at a fast rate.

After a big meal, your body puts out an excess of the fat-storage hormone insulin. Remember, extra insulin locks down the fat cell, inhibiting it from releasing fatty acids to be burned for energy. Eating smaller meals, and more often, is a lot like throwing logs on our slow-burning metabolic fires, getting them to burn better and brighter. It all starts with breakfast.

Don't think for a minute that you are wisely cutting calories or saving time by skipping breakfast. The truth is, those calories would be burned by your body's higher metabolic rate. You are only robbing your body of performance and metabolic fuel. And bypassing this morning metabolic boost doesn't affect just your weight, it can also affect your thinking abilities. Research has shown that missing breakfast can undercut reading skills and the ability to concentrate. A recent breakfast study showed a full letter grade differential in children who had breakfast compared with those who did not. Not only that, the study reported a poorer attitude and behavior problems among the children who missed breakfast. A study at the University of Wales found that breakfast-skippers were less able than breakfast-eaters to recall a word list and a story that was read aloud to them.

Because breakfast stabilizes your blood chemistries, you will have more energy and alertness. It allows you to be more productive and effective, allowing you to do what you do quickly and more enjoyably—with fewer mistakes. How's that for a time investment?

But Breakfast Is a Pain!

Actually, people skip breakfast for lots of reasons. Again, some skip it to save calories, others skip it to save time. Some can't face food in the morning, and others just don't like breakfast foods.

If you are not hungry in the morning, it's more than likely

because your body has gone through some chemical gymnastics while you've slept, and you may wake up in a state of "morning sickness." It's not that you aren't in need of breakfast—just the opposite. Breakfast will neutralize your blood sugars and stomach acids and make you feel better.

A quite common reason for skipping breakfast is that in some people it seems to start a vicious appetite machine, making them hungry every few hours. If this is you, be assured that breakfast is not the problem; you get hungry soon after you've eaten breakfast because you take yourself out of the starved mode and raise your blood sugars. When you starve your body in the morning, the resulting use of your own tissue for energy releases waste products (ketones) into your system that temporarily depress your appetite and give you a feeling of fullness. You can continue to starve for many hours without feeling hunger.

CAN'T I JUST EAT A BREAKFAST BAR?

There is a wide variety of bars are available, from grain-and-"fruit" bars to granola or chocolate-covered bars pegged as meal replacements.

Although there is certainly nothing "wrong" with these products, we are probably misleading ourselves if we say they are an equal substitute for a balanced breakfast.

Most breakfast bars provide less fiber than you would get from a whole-grain cereal or toast, and most contain substantially more sugar than you might realize. (Check the label for sugar content. Remember that every four grams of sugar equals a teaspoonful.) Even products marketed as containing fruit really contain what is more like sugar-filled jam.

Perhaps heading to bed fifteen minutes earlier would allow you to get up with five minutes to spare for a breakfast that includes a more balanced selection of whole grains, proteins, and fruit without too much of a fat and sugar load. Even if you prefer dinner leftovers to traditional "breakfast foods," the key is the balance—and real foods, not packaged pep.

Sadly, this backfires later in the day. As soon as you begin to eat, the appetite really turns on, and you eat too much, too late. In addition, you've let your body go into a slowed metabolic state. Not only will you overeat because your blood sugar level has fallen so low, but, like the campfire, your body will not be able to burn those calories well. Remember, your body just cannot handle such a large intake of food at one time; your needs go on twenty-four hours a day.

In matters of nutrition, I talk a lot about investment and returns. Breakfast calories are a good example of this. The return is greater than the initial deposit because remaining calories eaten during the day burn more efficiently instead of being stored as fat. A Vanderbilt University study showed that overweight breakfast-skippers who started to eat breakfast lost an average of seventeen pounds in twelve weeks. Not only did eating breakfast speed up their metabolisms, it also caused them to be less hungry the rest of the day. Because they were eating the right foods at the right times, they were less apt to eat the wrong things at the wrong times.

The bottom line: Eat breakfast soon after you get up—within the first half-hour of arising—and have three different foods for breakfast: a quick, energy-starting simple carbohydrate (fruit), a long-lasting whole-grain complex carbohydrate (grains, cereals, bread, or muffins), and a power-building protein (dairy, egg, soy, or meat). This good-for-you balance will allow a slow and steady release of glucose into your bloodstream to feed your brain and muscles with vital energy. Selecting whole foods, rather than a Danish and fruit punch, also gives your body the vitamins and minerals it needs to transform the energy nutrients into usable fuel.

Go light and easy if time is a push; try some eat-and-go meals like fresh fruit and skim-milk shakes, cheese-toast and fruit, or freshly fruited yogurt with a muffin. And don't be concerned if the meals are not made up of traditional breakfast-food choices. Some nonbreakfast food-lovers start their day with a turkey or tuna sandwich or even a cheese quesadilla.

You may want to try the breakfast recipes on page 169—quick meals designed to give you the perfect start to an energy-filled day.

Eat Often

Once you start your day with breakfast, the goal is to keep your metabolic system and blood chemistries working for you. To prevent your blood sugar level from dropping and to keep your metabolic rate high, you need food distributed evenly throughout the day. Going many hours between meals causes the body to slow metabolically so that the next meal is perceived as an overload. Even if the meal is balanced and healthy, the nutrients cannot be used optimally—again, it's too much too late. And the lowered blood sugar will leave you sleepy and craving sweets. Snacking on the right foods is much more fun—and a lot more healthy.

This is what I call "power snacking"—eating the right amounts of the right foods at regular intervals—and it's an important component of The Smart Weigh.

The Slimming Secrets of Snacking

You may be thinking, "But I thought I wasn't supposed to eat between meals." Wrong! When most people think of snacks, they picture potato chips, candy, and sodas. These types of snacks are "empty calories," providing high amounts of fats, sugars, salt, and calories, but few or no vitamins or minerals. A healthy snack, on the other hand, provides you with real nutrition and will keep your blood sugar levels from dropping too low. It will keep your metabolism burning high, your needs satisfied.

Your daily eating should consist of three meals with at least two healthy snacks. Ideally, eat 25 percent of your day's calories at breakfast, 25 percent at lunch, 25 percent at dinner, and the other 25 percent in healthy snacks, eaten about every two and a half to three hours. This is not mindless grazing, which has been shown not to raise your metabolism; instead, it is eating strategically to go for the caloric burn. On average, weight loss winners eat five times a day.

Wise snacking will also invigorate your mind. Tests have shown that a snack eaten fifteen minutes before skill tests of memory, alertness, reading, or problem-solving greatly increased performance in test subjects, whereas those individuals who had eaten breakfast and lunch, but no snack, scored lower.

Iron-willed discipline has never controlled food intake and never will. No checklist or rigid diet plan will give that control. Wisely chosen foods and well-timed eating together are much more powerful and energizing. Strategic eating is essentially a balancing act, achieved by giving your body the right foods at the right time, and put together in effective ways. This means having both carbohydrates and proteins at every meal and snack, and keeping your healthy snack handy. When you don't have good choices available, you're likely to reach for an unhealthy snack or not eat at all, with either alternative setting you up for a later disaster.

Consider the healthy power snack ideas chart on page 41, and start making them a regular part of your daily diet. Many power snacks do not require refrigeration, so keep them available in your car, in your desk drawer, in your briefcase—wherever you might find yourself at critical times. They can be as simple as fresh or dried fruit with low-fat cheese or yogurt, half a sandwich, or a trail mix of dry-roasted peanuts, sunflower seeds, and dried fruit.

Eat Balanced

Eating evenly throughout the day is not the only important factor in keeping your metabolism burning high and your body working well. Balancing your intake of carbohydrates and proteins is also vital to utilizing nutrients optimally. Every meal (and power snack) should include both whole food carbohydrates and lean proteins.

I know that this notion slaps every pop diet in the face; all quick-

POWER SNACKS

- Whole-grain crackers and low-fat cheese (like string cheese, part-skim mozzarella, soy cheese, or Laughing Cow Lite Cheese Wedges)
- Fresh fruit or small box of raisins and low-fat cheese
- Half of a lean turkey or chicken sandwich on whole grain bread
- Plain, nonfat yogurt blended with fruit or all-fruit jam, or Stonyfield Farms yogurt
- Whole grain cereal with skim milk
- Wasa bread with light cream cheese and all-fruit jam
- Baked low-fat tortilla chips with fat-free bean dip and salsa
- Health Valley graham crackers or rice cakes with natural peanut butter
- Popcorn sprinkled with Parmesan cheese
- Homemade low-fat bran muffin with low-fat or skim milk
- Crisp bread with sliced turkey and Dijon mustard
- Small pop-top can of water-packed tuna or chicken with whole-grain crackers
- Half of a small, whole-wheat bagel or English muffin with 2 tablespoons light cream cheese
- Veggie tortilla rolls: whole-wheat tortilla spread with mustard or low-fat mayonnaise, and sprinkled with a variety of shredded vegetables, and 2 ounces low-fat grated cheese
- Fruit shake: skim milk blended with frozen fruit and vanilla
- Trail mix: 1 cup unsalted dry roasted peanuts or soy nuts, 1 cup unsalted dry roasted shelled pumpkin or sunflower seeds, and 2 cups raisins (make it in abundance and bag up into $\frac{1}{4}$ cup or $\frac{1}{2}$ cup portions for a whole snack)

weight-loss plans manipulate and throw off this balance to force quick weight loss from dehydration. But the only way to lose body fat without losing your health is to embrace balance. It's this balance that produces the metabolic burn we are seeking the most. In a study published in 1999, researchers found that healthy young women burned almost 50 percent more of their daily caloric intake when they ate meals that were low in fat and high in carbohydrates (with proper protein balance) than they did when eating meals that were lower in carbs but higher in fat.

Remember, carbohydrates and protein have very different functions in your body. Proteins are the vital building blocks for the body. Carbohydrates are 100 percent pure energy—your body's fuel, designed to burn fast, clean, and pure. When carbohydrates are eaten alone, the body uses them like kindling on a fire. It burns brightly and quickly, but the body-building functions of protein do not take place. While protein can be used as an energy source, it has another much more vital function, which is why carbohydrates should be eaten with a protein to protect this building nutrient from being wasted as a less efficient source of energy. This allows protein to be used for building new cells, boosting your metabolism, building body muscle, keeping body fluids in balance, healing and fighting infections, and making skin, hair, and nails beautiful.

Women generally need at least 50 to 55 grams of protein per day; men generally need 65 to 70 grams (these estimates are based on percentage of lean body mass). More protein is needed in times of stress, or when actively working to build muscle or to maintain muscle mass while losing fat weight. Generally, one ounce of meat contains about 7 grams of protein, meaning women need a minimum of 7 to 8 ounces per day and men need a minimum of 9 to 10 ounces per day. Generally, your power snacks should include at least 1 to 2 ounces of protein, and your meals should provide 2 to 3 ounces (after cooking). If possible, get a food scale and periodically weigh your protein portion to be sure you are getting enough.

But the amount of protein eaten is not the only secret to abundant energy and wellness; equally important is the need to take in protein in smaller, evenly distributed amounts throughout the day. Because protein is not stored, it must be replenished frequently throughout the day, each and every day. And this is where people go wrong. Never, never believe anybody who tells you that you don't need protein, or to eat it only once a day. You will be robbing your body of protein's healing and building power all day long.

POWER PROTEINS

Anything that comes from an animal (poultry, fish, meat, eggs, cheese, milk, and yogurt) gives you complete protein, supplying all the essential amino acids that your body can't make or store. The only plant source of quality protein, a miraculous one, is the legume family (dried beans and peanuts). Their pods absorb nitrogen from the soil and become an excellent high-fiber, low-fat protein source. Yet, because they lack sufficient amounts of one or more of the essential amino acids, they are considered "incomplete" proteins. They are best eaten with a grain (corn, wheat, rice, or oat product) or a seed (sunflower, sesame, pumpkin) to be complete.

Examples of high-quality dynamic duos are: peanut butter on bread, black beans over rice, beans and tortillas or cornbread, or a peanut and sunflower seed trail mix. Generally a $\frac{1}{2}$ cup of cooked beans serves as two ounces of protein when mixed with an appropriate grain or seed, and $\frac{3}{4}$ cup equals three ounces of protein.

Each of the following equals 1 ounce (7 grams) of protein:

- 6 ounces nonfat milk or nonfat plain yogurt
- 1 ounce or $\frac{1}{4}$ cup grated low-fat cheeses
- $\frac{1}{4}$ cup 1 percent low-fat or nonfat cottage cheese or part-skim or fat-free ricotta
- 1 egg (particularly egg white)
- 1 ounce or $\frac{1}{4}$ cup flaked fish, i.e., tuna, salmon
- $\frac{1}{4}$ cup crab, lobster
- 5 pieces clams, shrimp, oysters, scallops
- 1 ounce or $\frac{1}{4}$ cup chopped poultry
- 1 ounce beef, pork, lamb, veal (lean, trimmed)
- $\frac{1}{4}$ cup legumes (black, red, garbanzo, Great Northern, kidney, navy beans; lentils; peanuts; soybeans; split peas)
- 8 ounces soy products (such as tofu or soy milk)
- 2 tablespoons natural peanut butter

The bottom line: Be sure to eat proteins and carbs together. At every meal and power snack have a balance of high-quality, whole-food carbohydrate and lean proteins. Always remember:

ENERGY-BOOSTING CARBOHYDRATES

Carbohydrates are found in plant foods (wheat, corn, oats, rice, barley, fruits, and vegetables), and are nutrition heavyweights themselves. When chosen in their whole food forms, they are packed with fiber, vitamins, and minerals that allow your body to stay operative from a point of strength. Contrary to what you may have heard, carbohydrates are low in calories. It's what we cook them in or top them with (butter, mayonnaise, heavy oils, and dressing) that moves us into weight-gaining territory.

Some carbohydrates are digested and absorbed quite easily, allowing them to be quick-burning forms of energy. These are the simple carbohydrates, found in fruits, unsweetened juices, and crunchy vegetables. The closer the food is to how it is grown, the slower will be the release of its sugars into the bloodstream. Complex carbohydrates, found in root vegetables, legumes, and grains that have not been processed and refined, require more time to convert into a usable form of energy; they are digested more slowly and absorbed more evenly into the system as fuel. An eating plan high in whole-food forms of carbohydrates is your best bet for living long and well.

SIMPLE CARBOHYDRATES

Fruits: All fruits and fruit juices like apples, apricots, bananas, berries, cherries, dates, grapefruit, grapes, kiwis, lemons, limes, melons, nectarines, oranges, peaches, pears, pineapples, plums, raisins (Generally one serving of

---

Carbohydrates burn and proteins build. You need them both.

Best-Choice Carbohydrates

When choosing carbohydrates, go for the most whole form possible and thus benefit from all the fiber, nutrients, and natural chemicals they were created with. This means eating fruits and vegetables with well-washed skins on, and choosing fruit rather than fruit juice. Choose whole grains when you can, such as brown rice and stone-ground, 100 percent whole-grain breads, crackers, pastas, and cereals. Look for the word WHOLE as the first ingredient on the label. These foods supply much-needed vitamin B6, chromium, selenium, and magnesium—all nutrients that are critical for activating energy

simple carboyhdrates is obtained from ½ cup fruit, ½ cup fruit juice, or ⅛ cup dried fruit. This gives 10 grams of carbohydrates)

Nonstarchy Vegetables: asparagus, beets, broccoli, Brussels sprouts, cabbage, carrots, cauliflower, celery, green beans, green leafy vegetables, kale, mushrooms, okra, onions, snow peas, sugar snap peas, summer squash, tomatoes, zucchini (Generally one serving of simple carbohydrates is obtained from ½ cup cooked vegetables or 1 cup raw vegetables or juice—this gives 10 grams of simple carbohydrates)

COMPLEX CARBOHYDRATES

Grains: The following amounts provide one serving of complex carbohydrates, giving 15 grams: ½ cup cooked barley, bulgur, couscous, grits, kasha, millet, or polenta; 1 slice bread; 1 ounce cereal (¼ cup of concentrated cereal such as Grape Nuts or granola, ½ to ¾ cup flaked cereals, 1 cup puffed cereal); 1 cup crackers or 5 mini-rice cakes; 2 crispbread or rice cakes; ⅓ cup oats, uncooked; ½ cup pasta or rice, cooked; 1 fat-free tortilla; ¼ cup wheat germ

Starchy Vegetables: black-eyed peas, corn, green peas, lima beans, rutabagas, turnips, potatoes (white and sweet), winter squash (Generally one serving of complex carbohydrates is obtained from ½ cup cooked starchy vegetables, giving 15 grams)

production and release. They also have a lower glycemic response.

Whole-grain carbohydrates are particularly valuable because they have not had the outer layers of grain removed; they contain many more vitamins, minerals, and fiber than the refined, white products. Don't be fooled by manufacturers and advertisements. White, refined carbohydrates, even when enriched, are never as good nutritionally as whole grains. In fact, to your body, refined white flour is the same as sugar, making a diet high in white-flour foods the same as a high-sugar diet. Start reading the ingredients lists of all your grain products and remember to choose those made with 100 percent whole grain. Many manufacturers call products whole grain even if they contain only minimal amounts of bran. Brown dye does wonders in making food look healthy.

Whole grains satisfy and keep you full, so you may eat less in general. The fiber they contain slows the rate of nutrient absorption following a meal, reducing the rise of blood sugar levels and secretion of insulin that causes the fat cells to lock down. Fiber serves as a "time-release capsule," releasing sugars from digested carbohydrates slowly and evenly into the bloodstream. This helps keep your energy levels up and even.

Eat Lean

One of the drawbacks to eating more protein more often is that

FIBER: A POWERFUL WEIGHT-LOSS BOOSTER

Dietary fiber (the part of plants not digested by the body) promotes weight loss by helping to block the body's digestion of fat. A recent study of 3,700 men and women ages 18 to 30 showed that those who had the highest intakes of fiber-rich whole grains also tended to have lower body fat. The study showed that at all levels of fat intake, individuals eating the most fiber gained less weight than those eating the least fiber.

In another study, people absorbed fewer calories when the fiber content of their meals was increased. Individuals who upped their daily fiber intake from 18 grams to 36 grams (a bowl of high-fiber cereal can contain 25 grams) absorbed 130 fewer calories per day. Over the course of a year, that reduction in calorie uptake would bring a loss of roughly ten pounds.

There are two types of fiber: the water-soluble fibers found in oats, barley, apples, dried beans, and nuts, which have been found to lower serum cholesterol and triglyceride levels and to help control blood sugar levels; and the water-insoluble fibers found in wheat bran, whole grains, and fresh vegetables, which are excellent means of controlling chronic GI problems.

Think of fiber as a sponge that absorbs excess water in the GI tract to curtail diarrhea but provides a bulky mass which will pass more quickly and easily to relieve constipation and diverticulosis and possibly prevent hemorrhoids. Fiber many popular choices are also high in fat. But does fat make you fat? It's not quite that simple, but fat is more than just a disease culprit; excess intake is also a culprit in fat storage and metabolic lockdown. It's theorized that overeating fat sends fat molecules into your bloodstream, increasing the thickness, or viscosity, of the blood, and reducing its oxygen-delivery capacity. And it's the oxygen that's needed for energy to be metabolized rather than stored. In addition, the excess calories we consume as fat are converted and stored as fat more readily than those from other sources. One reason for this is that fat is a more concentrated source of calories, and all fats contain twice as many calories as equal amounts of carbohydrate or proteins, about 9 calories per gram, or 120 calories per tablespoon.

needs water to make it work the way it should, ideally 8 to 10 glasses a day. The best way to drink water is to have a glass before and after every meal and snack rather than with a meal when it dilutes digestive functions. Try filling a two-quart container with water each morning and make sure you have drunk it all before bedtime.

To increase the amount of fiber you get in your diet easily, choose more raw and lightly cooked vegetables but in as nonprocessed form as possible. As a food becomes processed, ground, mashed, puréed, or juiced, the fiber effectiveness is decreased. Add unprocessed raw bran to your cereals. Raw oat bran (from oatmeal) is particularly useful in stabilizing blood sugar and cholesterol levels; raw wheat bran is useful for a healthy gastrointestinal tract. Be careful to add bran gradually. Begin with 1 teaspoon wheat bran and 1 teaspoon oat bran and increase slowly as your body adjusts to more fiber.

High-Fiber Foods: Peanuts and peanut butter; Cooked dried beans; Sunflower and sesame seeds; Apples, apricots, peaches, pears, bananas, pineapple, plums, prunes; Broccoli, carrots, corn, lettuce, peas, potatoes (including skins), spinach; Bran (unprocessed wheat and oat); Bread (whole wheat); Brown rice; Cereals (whole grain, bran type, oatmeal, Wheatena); Whole-wheat pasta

Also, the body is more efficient in storing fat as fat. This is why the weight control experts of today consider "trimming the fat" from our diets to be much more important in weight loss than just watching our calories.

Of course, fatness or thinness is not the only issue involved in our food choices. Even if you have been blessed with a metabolism that burns ever brightly, allowing you to maintain your weight easily, excess fat intake can bring problems. You may not be seeing the problem, on the scale or on your waistline, but it's an energy drain and a disease flag just the same.

Intriguing research on fat's effect on our metabolism has come out of Duke University, showing that type II diabetic mice put on a radically reduced fat intake diet (10 percent of total calories consumed) were cured of their diabetes. This reflects the impact that an excess fat intake can have on blood sugar levels—of both mice and men. It also makes a statement about the risk of diets that push fat and radically cut valuable carbohydrates as a diabetes cure. The truth is that excess fat fed to animals with a genetic susceptibility to diabetes made them far more likely to develop the disease.

And there's more. Look at these vital facts about fat:

- Excess fat intake increases your cholesterol level and your risk of heart disease and stroke.
- Excess fat intake increases your risk of cancer.
- Excess fat intake, particularly saturated fat, has been shown to elevate blood pressure, regardless of your weight or sodium intake.

The bottom line: Choose your proteins wisely by making them low-fat. You certainly do need fat; it is an essential nutrient needed in limited amounts to lubricate your body, transport fat-soluble vitamins, produce hormones, and fill you after eating. But it needs to come from the healthiest sources, not from bacon fat and butter.

Cutting calories is easier if you focus on limiting fat to less than 30 percent of daily calories. Cutting back on calories from fat allows you to eat more nutrient-rich foods like whole grains, fruits, and vegetables. You can also eat more food for fewer calories.

Determining Your Personal Fat Budget

As much as we need a balancing act of carbohydrates and proteins at each meal, we don't need fat in the quantities we consume. On average, too much of our calorie intake is from fat—35 to 40 percent rather than the recommended 25 to 30 percent. The typical adult eats the fat equivalent of one stick of butter a day. Even if you don't eat that much fat, chances are you are eating a lot more than you realize.

To really understand your fat limit, you need to know your calorie limit. To lose weight, a moderately active woman will probably need to keep her daily caloric intake to around 1,500 calories. A moderately active man shouldn't exceed around 1,800 calories. To determine your 25 percent fat allowance, use this formula:

25 percent of 1,500 calories = 375 calories

375 calories divided by 9 calories per gram of fat = 42 grams of total fat suggested each day.

Once you know your fat budget, see whether you are staying within the bounds by adding up the grams of fat for all the food that you eat in a day. This is both the fat hidden in foods you eat—the fat in chicken, fish, and cheese—as well as the added fat you cook with or add to your food, like oils or butter. Almost all food labels will tell you the grams of total fat in a serving.

Like any worthy goal, reducing your personal fat intake requires some effort and commitment—to learn new ways to season foods without fat, to order more healthfully at restaurants, to discover the right snack foods. Be assured that the benefits far exceed the effort. Smart eating does not doom you to nutrition martyrdom—eating flavorless foods that taste like cardboard. Nor do you have to become a chemical analyst to stay within these guidelines while dining out, grocery shopping, or cooking. Use the Real-Life Strategies in Part 2 to help you trim the fat without cutting flavor.

Think of a move toward nutritious, low-fat eating as a permanent change instead of a dieting regimen that you go on and go off. Don't keep a calculator at your bedside, and don't get stuck in a deprivation mode. Be easy on yourself, and go slowly, taking practical, feasible steps one at a time. Focus on good foods, well prepared, and your desires will begin to shift. Give your taste buds time to return to how they were created; high-fat foods will have less and less appeal as you begin to eat foods that kick up your metabolism and give you energy, better digestion, and a sense of well-being.

If motivation to cut back on the fat in your diet comes hard, consider this mental picture: Imagine hamburger grease after it cools and hardens. Then imagine that grease trying to circulate through your bloodstream.

ALL ABOUT OIL

We eat five kinds of oil: saturated, hydrogenated, polyunsaturated, monounsaturated, and omega-3 fatty acids. Each has the same fat content and number of calories that contribute to the fat budget: 5 grams of fat and 45 calories per teaspoon.

But these oils vary greatly in the effects they have on our bodies—good and bad. Some are damaging to the arteries and heart.

ARTERY-CLOGGING FATS THAT INCREASE BLOOD CHOLESTEROL:

Saturated fat: Found in dairy and meat products, including milk, cheese, ice cream, beef, and pork. It also can be found in coconut and palm oils, nondairy creamers, and toppings.

Hydrogenated fat: Also called trans fat, hydrogenated fat is formed when vegetable oils are hardened into solids, usually to protect against spoiling and to maintain flavor. Examples include stick margarine and shortening, deep-fried foods such as French fries and fried chicken, and pastries, cookies, doughnuts, and crackers. Read the ingredient list of any processed foods you buy. If you see the words "partially hydrogenated," look for a different product—especially if it is one of the first three ingredients. Hydrogenation is a manufacturing process that converts a polyunsaturated or monounsaturated oil into a saturated fat.

Eat Bright

Brightly colored fruits and vegetables are loaded with antioxidants like beta-carotene and vitamin A, folic acid, and other B vitamins, along with vitamin C. These nutrients are vital to wellness since they neutralize chemicals believed to damage body processes and serve to boost metabolism by boosting the immune system.

A good way to picture the immune system is as a disciplined and effective personal "border patrol," with soldiers and scouts on permanent duty throughout your body. These warriors include several different types of white blood cells, each with its own special mission. Together they work to identify a threat to the body, call an alert, and divide into army battalions to attack the enemy and stabilize the body. It all happens so quickly, you often don't even know you were threatened. But to keep your border patrol officers alert

---

FATS THAT DO NOT CLOG ARTERIES INCLUDE:

Monounsaturated fat: Found in olive, canola, and peanut oils. These fats increase good HDL cholesterol and decrease bad LDL cholesterol, and thus the risk of disease.

Omega-3 Fatty Acids (EPA and DHA Oils): Found in all fish and seafood, particularly cold-water fish such as salmon, albacore tuna, swordfish, sardines, mackerel, and hard shellfish. The only significant plant source is flaxseed. Omega-3 fatty acids decrease triglycerides and total and bad LDL cholesterol. They reduce the tendency of the blood to form clots, stabilize blood sugars, improve brain function, and reduce inflammation.

Polyunsaturated fats decrease both bad LDL and good HDL cholesterol, so they aren't the desired choice. These fats are those in corn oil, cottonseed oil, safflower oil, sesame oil, sunflower oil, as well as avocado, sunflower seed kernels, sesame seeds, almonds, walnuts, and pecans.

Try to get most of your fat from monounsaturated olive and canola oil (or salad dressings made from them), nuts, and the omega-3s found in fish and flaxseed. And spread your fat throughout the day—a little fat helps you absorb fat-soluble nutrients from vegetables and fruit.

and strong, the immune system needs to be kept fit and fueled, mobilized for action.

And that's where fruits and vegetables come in. Generally, the more vivid the color of the fruit or veggie, the higher in nutrients it will be. The bright color signals that these are treasure chests of protection, and triggers for releasing energy and raising immunities.

That deep orange-red color of carrots, sweet potatoes, apricots, cantaloupe, and strawberries is a sign of their vitamin A content. Dark green leafy vegetables like greens, spinach, romaine lettuce, broccoli, and Brussels sprouts, also have the extra bonus of being the source of folic acid (folate), a must-have for health and wellness. The presence of folate in the blood seems to lower the level of homocysteine, an amino acid that may be a cause of stroke and

> ## TIPS TO RETAIN NUTRIENTS
>
> - Buy vegetables that are as fresh as possible. When not possible, frozen is the next best choice. Avoid those frozen with butter or sauces.
> - Use well-washed peelings and outer leaves of vegetables whenever possible because of the high concentration of nutrients found within them.
> - Store vegetables in airtight containers in the refrigerator.
> - Do not store vegetables in water. Too many vitamins are lost.
> - Cook vegetables on the highest heat possible, in the least amount of water possible, and for the shortest time possible. Steaming, microwaving, and stir-frying are the best cooking methods.
> - Cook vegetables until tender crisp, not mushy. Overcooked vegetables lose their flavor along with their vitamins.

heart disease. A variety of foods contain folate, including breakfast cereals as well as beans and green vegetables. Since January 1998 the federal government has insisted that folate be added to all flour. So it's in your bread, whether you eat it sliced, wrapped, or by the baguette.

Without trying to calculate every milligram of this vitamin and that mineral in the foods you eat, the best way to assure that your vitamin intake is optimal is to go for whole-grain carbohydrates whenever possible, and choose meals full of a variety of brightly colored fruits and vegetables.

The ideal is nine servings of vegetables and fruits every day. Veggies and fruit are the foundation of The Smart Weigh plan, as opposed to grains, the foundation of the traditional food pyramid. You should be eating nine ½ cup servings (about 4½ cups) of a variety of brightly colored fruits and veggies every day.

Sound like overkill? In reality, it could spell extra life. Study after study links diets highest in fruit and vegetables with less cancer, heart disease, diabetes, even osteoporosis. The landmark DASH (Dietary Approaches to Stop Hypertension) diet study found that nine servings a day lowered high blood pressure as much as some prescription drugs. More and more research suggests that nine a day—five vegetables and four fruits—is the optimum. Yet most Americans get only four servings a day.

Antioxidant Power

For fifty years or so, a leading hypothesis has been that aging and disease are promoted by highly reactive molecules called free radicals. The older we get, the more free radicals are released into our systems, where they destroy tissue. The villain is oxygen. In effect, we rust as we get older! But the body also has a network of defenses against free radicals, called antioxidants. Some are produced internally; others are derived from what we eat.

Vitamin E is one such antioxidant. Many other antioxidants also promise protection against diseases. One is lutein, found in leafy green vegetables, which may help protect against degeneration of the macula in the eye, the leading cause of blindness in those sixty-five or older. Another is lycopene, contained in tomatoes, apricots, guava, pink grapefruit, and watermelon, which may help prevent prostate cancer. And exciting beneficial effects are being shown through the antioxidants contained in red wine, blueberries, and strawberries as well.

As the research continues to pour in, this is the best health insurance policy: nine servings a day of brightly colored fruits and vegetables will help to keep the doctor away...and ten servings will allow you to thrive, especially if complemented with other antioxidant-rich foods such as garlic, hot peppers, green tea, and soy.

Food Heals

A discussion about strategic eating wouldn't be complete without some comments on the pharmacological wonders of food. If you have been eating foods just to lose weight or just because it's dinner time, you are missing an important and exciting truth: Food is filled with healing agents, like the antioxidants mentioned above, that energize and power you. Food is medicine for your body.

If you desire to get well, stay well, and live a life filled with energy, you must expose your body to food because of what's in food: natural healing agents, mood enhancers, and energy boosters. There are certain foods that pack a powerful punch when it comes to wellness. In addition to their wealth of vitamins and minerals, these foods contain

EAT LIKE THE GREEKS!

A Mediterranean diet may help protect people against rheumatoid arthritis, Greek investigators report. Study findings published in the American Journal of Clinical Nutrition from the University of Athens Medical School show that a high intake of cooked vegetables and olive oil may reduce the risk of developing the disease.

The research team compared the diets of 145 rheumatoid arthritis patients with the diets of 188 people who did not have the disease. All of the study participants lived in southern Greece, where the average diet consists of less meat and more cooked and raw vegetables, fish, and olive oil than most diets in Westernized countries. Participants who ate the greatest number of servings of cooked vegetables were about 75 percent less likely to develop rheumatoid arthritis than those who reported eating the fewest servings. People with the lowest intake of cooked vegetables ate 0.85 servings of cooked vegetables a day, on average, and people with the highest intakes ate an average of 2.9 half-cup servings a day.

nutraceuticals, the food pharmacy for the new millennium.

This may be a new thought for you. Most of us are much more aware of the food/*disease* connection: if a person has diabetes, refined sugar is a bad thing; if he's allergic to shellfish, eating lobster is a bad thing; if she has high cholesterol, saturated fat is a *very* bad thing. Yet most people are just becoming aware of the food/*wellness* connection. And it's the most exciting part of health research today—a focus on the essential building blocks in food that make us well and keep us well.

This new perspective takes us beyond Mom's chiding to "eat your vegetables" because they're good for us. Instead, it's an understanding of what in broccoli makes it exciting to eat—indoles and sulforaphanes that protect against cancer and aging, folic acid that protects against heart disease, and vitamin C that boosts immune responses.

These truths are why I'm a "food pusher." This perspective builds appreciation and awe for lycopene in tomatoes—the antioxidant mentioned above that strongly protects against prostate and cervical cancer. Or for the b-glucan in whole oats that does medical magic by reducing cholesterol levels, increasing protection from cancer, regulating blood sugars, and serving as a gastrointestinal stabilizer.

The foods in my "Nutritional Top Ten" list can make all the difference. Review this list, and then review your food choices over the past week. How are you measuring up? It may be time to go to the grocery store and to start saying yes, not yuck, to power foods for your body.

There are so many other foods that could be placed on this Nutritional Top Ten list, some that may surprise you—like blueberries as a potent anti-ager and green tea as a brew for a slimmer you. That's right, energy expenditure scientists in Switzerland have found that the flavonoid in green tea—epigallocatechin galate (EGCG)—has been found to "turn up the burn" in fat oxidation, helping the body to better burn body fat rather than store it. If you must turn to caffeine for an energy hit, turn to green tea instead of espresso.

THE NUTRITIONAL TOP TEN

1. Oats: The b-glucan in whole oats reduces the risk of coronary heart disease. The soluble fiber is instrumental in lowering cholesterol and stabilizing blood sugars.

2. Soybeans: The bioactive ingredients in soy products suppress formation of blood vessels that feed cancer cells. Soy helps stabilize hormone levels in women, as well as decrease the risk of heart disease, osteoporosis, and ovarian, breast, and prostate cancers.

3. Tomatoes: Lycopene, a potent antioxidant, is a carotenoid that fights the uncontrolled growth of cells into tumors. It fights cancer of the colon, bladder, pancreas, and prostate. Men who eat ten servings of tomatoes per week have been shown to decrease their prostate cancer risk by 66 percent.

4. Cold-water seafood: Healthy EPA/omega-3 oils are shown to turn on fat oxidation, decrease risk of coronary artery disease, stabilize blood sugars, increase brain power, and reduce the inflammatory response. Seafood reduces LDL cholesterol and triglycerides, while raising levels of HDL cholesterol.

5. Flaxseed: A unique source of lignans, powerful antioxidants that are believed to stop cells from turning cancerous. Flaxseed also contains alpha-linolenic acid, the plant version of the omega-3s found in fish oils; it makes a great healthy option for people who don't eat fish.

6. Garlic: Rich in allicin, which boosts immune function and reduces cancer

---

What About Vitamins and Minerals?

Vitamins and essential minerals are required in tiny amounts to promote essential biochemical reactions in your cells. Together, vitamins and minerals are called micronutrients. Lack of a particular micronutrient for a prolonged period can cause a specific disease or condition, which can usually be reversed when the micronutrient is resupplied.

A vitamin deficiency takes you down over time. It may take months, but it's a slow decline into fatigue and weakness. As your body becomes depleted of certain vitamins, various biochemical changes take place that result in a general lack of well-being. This occurs long before any symptoms of a specific vitamin deficiency can be noted. For risk. Garlic also has strong antiviral effects and has been shown to lower blood pressure and cholesterol levels.

7. Hot peppers: A source of capsaicin, a vital immune, mood, and metabolic booster with powerful antiviral effects. Capsaicin is linked to decreased risk of stomach cancer due to its ability to neutralize nitrosamines, a cancer-causing compound formed in the body when cured or charred meats are consumed. Capsaicin also kills bacteria believed to cause stomach ulcers, and appears to turn on the fat-burning capacity.

8. Sweet potatoes: A rival of carrots as a potent source of beta-carotene and other carotenoids, which help prevent cataracts and protect the body from free radicals and cancer—particularly cancer of the larynx, esophagus, and lungs.

9. Grapes: Grape skins contain a high concentration of resveratrol, which appears to block the formation of coronary artery plaque, as well as tumor formation and growth. Red grape juice or red wine is considered a better source of resveratrol than white, which is made without the grape skins.

10. Cruciferous vegetables: Broccoli, cabbage, cauliflower, and Brussels sprouts contain indoles, sulforaphane, and isothiocyanates which protect cells from damage by carcinogens, block tumor formation, and help the liver to inactivate hormone-like compounds that may promote cancer.

example, a thiamine deficiency can ultimately exhibit itself as nerve damage, but appetite loss, weakness, and lethargy will precede it.

Your body can't make most vitamins and minerals. They must come from food or supplements. Vitamins are organic minerals that the body does not produce on its own but cannot do without. As chemical catalysts for the body, they make things happen. Although vitamins do not themselves give energy, they help the body convert carbohydrates to energy and then help the body to metabolize it.

There are thirteen vitamins. Four—vitamins A, D, E, and K—are stored in your body's fat (they're called fat-soluble vitamins). Nine are water-soluble and are not stored in your body in appreciable amounts. They are vitamin C and the eight B vitamins: thiamine

(B1), riboflavin (B2), niacin, vitamin B6, pantothenic acid, vitamin B12, biotin, and folic acid (folate).

In addition to their impact on your metabolism, vitamins in the right amounts are needed for normal growth, digestion, mental alertness, and resistance to infection. They enable your body to use carbohydrates, fats, and proteins. They also act as catalysts in your body, initiating or speeding up a chemical reaction. But you don't "burn" vitamins, so you can't get energy (calories) directly from them.

Your body strives to maintain an optimal level of each vitamin and keep a constant amount circulating in your bloodstream. Surplus water-soluble vitamins are excreted in urine. Surplus fat-soluble vitamins are stored in body tissue. Because they're stored, excess fat-soluble vitamins can accumulate in your body and become toxic. Your body is especially sensitive to too much vitamin A and vitamin D. For example, taking large amounts of vitamin D can indirectly cause kidney damage, and large amounts of vitamin A can cause liver damage. Even modest increases in some minerals can lead to imbalances that limit your body's ability to use other minerals. And supplements of iron, zinc, chromium, and selenium can be toxic at just five times the Daily Value, or DV. Megadose formulas can also cause stomach pains, diarrhea, and kidney stones. Virtually all nutrient toxicities stem from high-dose supplements—more is not necessarily better, and can even be harmful.

Minerals, unlike vitamins, are inorganic compounds. Some minerals are building blocks for the body structures such as bones and teeth. Others work with the fluids in the body, giving them certain characteristics. Some thirty minerals are important in nutrition, although most are needed only in small, yet vital, amounts.

Like an insufficient intake of vitamins, mineral deficiencies also zap your metabolism, particularly when there is a lack of the high-energy nutrients iron, magnesium, and zinc. Your body also needs fifteen minerals that help regulate cell function and provide structure for cells. Major minerals include calcium, phosphorus, and magne-

YOUR SUPPLEMENT GUIDE

Supplements are not substitutes. They can't replace the hundreds of nutrients in whole foods needed for a balanced diet. But if you do decide to take a vitamin supplement, here are things to consider:

Stick to the Daily Value: Choose a vitamin-mineral combination limited to 150 percent DV or less. Take no more than the recommended dose. The higher the dose, the more likely you are to have side effects.

Don't waste dollars: Generic brands and synthetic vitamins are generally less expensive and equally effective. Don't be tempted by added herbs, enzymes, or amino acids—they add nothing but cost. If you are going to use an herbal remedy, do that separately.

Read the label: Supplements can lose potency over time, so check the expiration date on the label. Also look for the initials USP (for the testing organization U.S. Pharmacopeia) or words such as "release assured" or "proven release," indicating that the supplement is easily dissolved and absorbed by your body.

Store them in a safe place: Iron supplements are a common cause of poisoning deaths among children. Keep them out of little hands' reach—and in a cool place.

Don't self-prescribe: See your doctor if you have a health problem. Tell him or her about any supplement you're taking. Some supplements may interfere with medications.

sium. In addition, your body needs smaller amounts of chromium, copper, fluoride, iodine, iron, manganese, molybdenum, selenium, zinc, chloride, potassium, and sodium.

Vitamin hucksters spend millions planting the fear: "Are you getting enough vitamins?" They recommend vitamin, mineral, and nutritional supplements as "vitamin insurance." But there's no need for most people to take out vitamin insurance. The American Dietetic Association, the National Academy of Sciences, the National Research Council, and other major medical societies all agree that as your first choice you should get the vitamins and minerals you need through a well-balanced diet. Although certain high-risk groups may benefit from a vitamin-mineral supplement, healthy adults can get all necessary nutrients from food. But most people don't.

And they don't for a reason different from what you might think: It's not a nutrient deficiency of our food supply, it's that most people don't eat properly. Only one person in ten, for example, regularly consumes the recommended five to nine servings of fruits and vegetables per day. Skipping meals, dieting, and eating meals high in sugar and fat all contribute to poor nutrition. For these people, taking supplemental vitamins would be reasonable and wise, although the best course would be to adopt better eating habits.

Food is better than supplements because food contains hundreds of additional nutrients, including phytochemicals. As already discussed, phytochemicals are compounds that occur naturally in foods containing important health benefits. Scientists have yet to learn all the roles phytochemicals play in nutrition, and there's no DV yet established for them. But this is known: If you depend on supplements rather than trying to eat a variety of whole foods, you miss out on possible health benefits from these natural protectors. In addition, only long-term, well-designed studies can sort out which nutrients in food are beneficial and whether taking them in pill form provides the same benefit. In the meantime, it's best to concentrate on getting your nutrients from food.

But it is admittedly difficult to get enough of some vitamins from the most conscientious diet. Vitamin E, for example, in high dosages may help prevent some cancers and cardiovascular disease. To get that much from your diet, you'd have to consume 1½ quarts of olive oil a day! Overall, however, it is better if your vitamin sources come from natural food rather than supplementation. But a cautionary note: The full benefits of a high dosage of vitamin E are not yet proved. In fact, still troublesome research reports are cropping up showing that antioxidant supplementation can actually trigger cancer cell growth and depress immune function.

The most intelligent course is to get the maximum vitamin and mineral intake you can from food, then use supplements. If you choose to take a multivitamin mineral supplement, look for one that has no more than 150 percent of the DV. Name-brand multivitamins sold at pharmacies are fine.

And be aware that a multivitamin mineral supplement will not fully meet your needs for certain nutrients like calcium and it will never be a substitute for food. The additional supplements I most commonly recommend are: 100 to 400 international units (IU) of vitamin E and 100 to 500 milligrams (mg) of vitamin C. On days when you may eat only two calcium-rich foods, take 500 mg of calcium if you're under fifty; take 1,000 mg of calcium (divided into two separate doses of 500 mg each) if you're fifty or older. Calcium citrate has been found to be the most absorbable supplement form.

The bottom line: If you want to improve your nutritional health, look first to a well-balanced diet. In most cases, making changes in your diet has a far greater chance of promoting health than taking supplements.

The beautiful thing about good, balanced nutrition is this: Everything fits together in such a perfect way that just eating a wide variety of different foods in their whole form will more than likely give you an adequate intake of essential nutrients. Eating well is the time-tested answer to the vitamin-mineral question, so don't let a junk diet vandalize your metabolism and energy stores any longer. Determine to make changes for the long haul. Learn how to eat and live with it for the rest of your life.

Eating to boost your metabolism and wellness has another payoff: It energizes you to exercise! Eating smart is only half the battle in your quest for an active metabolism—regular exercise is also a key to keeping your body burning calories at a high rate.

CHAPTER 4

S

MOVEMENT

A

R

T

EXERCISE IS CRITICAL TO LOSING weight and keeping it off. In fact, it's the single best predictor of whether you'll keep excess pounds off once you've lost them. A study done in Boston over a decade ago showed that people who dieted to lose weight but did not exercise gained back nearly all their weight, but those who exercised along with dieting, and continued to do so, didn't regain any.

This is primarily because of the impact exercise has on muscle mass. When you start using muscle during exercise rather than losing it to dieting, you release your fat-burning potential. Strong muscles are a lot like the Energizer Bunny: They just keep going and going, activating your metabolism and boosting your calorie burn even while you sleep. New research shows that by building muscle, you can further boost the calorie burn you get out of any kind of exercise.

You probably know that the amount of calories that you burn during exercise depends on what type of exercise you do, your level of effort, and how much you weigh. Yet when researchers at the Human

Performance and Fitness Department at the University of Massachusetts compared bodybuilders who had lots of muscle and little fat with men of the same weight who had less muscle and more fat, they found that the bodybuilders burned about 100 calories more during the same thirty-minute walk. They theorize that the good news will hold true for anyone building muscle, in any amount. Strong muscles rev up the body's calorie-burning ability. That is why exercise, particularly strength training, is the anti-aging solution. Lifting weights curbs muscle loss—along with shaping a sleeker, firmer body.

Aerobic (meaning "with oxygen") exercise is a powerful metabolic enhancer because it boosts the oxygen-carrying capacity of the bloodstream. During aerobic exercise, your heart pumps more blood, your lungs take in more oxygen, and your blood carries more oxygen and fuel to your muscles. The glucose from your food combines with oxygen in your cells, producing and releasing the energy molecules you need for a fast-burning metabolism. This means exercise gives you more metabolic-boosting oxygen where you need it, faster, and more efficiently. And by making your heart more efficient in its function, aerobic exercise improves brain circulation and function as well.

In addition to increasing your caloric burn while you're running the track or pedaling the stationary bike, exercise is a gift that keeps on giving. The "afterburn" of exercise boosts your metabolism so you use up more calories for hours after you finish your workout. This is the real impact of exercise and is especially beneficial if you exercise at higher rather than lower intensities—walking, running, or riding just a little faster, or adding some hills or incline to crank up the calorie burn and keep it up, even after your workout.

Exercise also decreases your appetite and gives you a healthy outlet for stress. It douses the emotional fires behind overeating. Endorphins—the powerful morphine-like chemicals that promote a sense of well-being—are also released in your brain during exercise. And moderate regular exercise can create a change in biochemistry that launches you into a state of confidence and exhilaration. Studies have proved that just thirty minutes of aerobic activity—all at once or in three ten-minute spurts throughout the day—will boost your energy, moods, and alertness. The overall effect of consistent exercise is to provide you better fuel to work with and a better engine to put it in.

Yet most people don't exercise at all. Surveys show that only 40 percent of Americans are involved in any kind of focused exercise on even a weekly basis—which adds up to 40 to 50 million people.

Exercise Equals Energy

Why don't people exercise? I believe the answer is simple: Too many of us are stuck in a vicious cycle of exhaustion. We know we need to exercise, but we are simply too done in to get it done. That's why I usually develop a phased Smart Weigh plan for my clients, first getting them to eat well and to start easy walking. After two to three weeks, a more focused exercise plan will emerge as a result of the overflow of energy. With this dynamic duo, the exercise adds significantly to their energy level and a positive cycle replaces the negative, downward energy cycle.

When you feel too tired to get moving, keep reminding yourself of this: The fastest way to feel energized is to exercise. That "I'm too tired to work out" feeling will get out of your head once you start moving. You just have to override the message of your stressed-out brain and do something—anything—physical when you're in an energy slump. When you get home feeling totally beat, push yourself a bit: Change into sneakers and go out for a brisk walk. You'll feel a burst of energy afterward. Then the next time you're feeling too pooped to exercise, you'll remember that "buzz" and be quicker to get off the couch. You may even be inclined to expand your workout into a more ambitious run or bike ride, or even a visit to the gym. Soon you'll be healthfully hooked on the buzz of working out and won't even hear those "I'm just too tired" messages from your brain.

Not exercising is associated with an increased rate of illness and disease of nearly every type, from the common cold and flu to heart disease and stroke. People who don't exercise are more apt to die from cardiovascular incidents than to survive them. And because of the interconnected nature of the muscular system, brain, and other processes of the body, being sedentary also depresses your mood, your thinking, and your ability to work productively.

Here are fourteen motivators to get you going and keep you going:

1. You'll Live Longer. An apple a day may keep the doctor away, but a two-mile walk may keep the coroner at bay. Researchers at the Honolulu Heart Program found that adults who walked an average of two miles a day reduced their risk of premature death by half. For the subjects who walked even more, the risk of death fell even further.

2. You'll Burn Calories. Particularly when you walk. Researchers at the Medical College of Wisconsin and Veterans Affairs Medical Center in Milwaukee tested the calorie burn of six indoor exercise machines and found the treadmill burned the most. When study participants exercised "somewhat hard," they burned a full 40 percent more calories walking on the treadmill than when on the stationary bike.

3. You'll Give Your Back a Break. The best thing you can do for a painful lower back is to perform moderate, low-impact exercise, like walking thirty to forty minutes, three to five days a week. Just avoid hills (which stress your back) and use good technique. Stand up straight, and don't let your stomach stick out or your head droop down.

4. You'll Build Bone Mass and Slim Your Middle. Weight-bearing exercise like walking or weight-lifting promotes bone growth—a big plus in the battle against osteoporosis. And if you walk at a brisk clip (four mph), you may encourage your body to secrete more growth hormone, which strengthens bones and increases lean body mass.

5. You'll Feel Less Pain. Researchers at the University of Florida in Gainesville corralled sixteen brave volunteers willing to have their index fingers pinched for two minutes before and after thirty minutes of exercise, then again after thirty minutes of quiet time. Once they recovered the power of speech, all the volunteers reported that the pain was most bearable right after exercise.

6. You'll Neutralize Premenstrual Symptoms. Regular aerobic exercise like walking can tame even the worst premenstrual symptoms by raising the level of endorphins in the brain and by increasing your circulation, which helps minimize bloating.

7. You'll Get a Good Night's Sleep. A Stanford University study of forty-three men and women with mild insomnia revealed that those who walked briskly for thirty to forty minutes four times a week for four months slept almost an hour longer per night and fell asleep faster.

8. You'll Look Better. Regular exercise gets your blood as well as your body moving. This increased circulation transports nutrients to your skin and quickly flushes out waste products. This leaves your skin glowing with enhanced health.

9. You'll Outsmart Middle-Age Spread. You know it's true: Metabolism slows naturally with age, but not necessarily because of aging. The decline in metabolic rate over time has less to do with advancing age than with declining activity. A University of Colorado study revealed that middle-aged and older women who exercised regularly didn't experience the age-related decline in their resting metabolic rate as did their sedentary counterparts. As a result, they stayed thinner and healthier—despite their advancing age.

10. You'll Take Stress in Stride. When you're confronted with a stressful situation, your body prepares to fight or take flight, in part by secreting catecholamines, chemicals that raise your heart rate and blood pressure and pump blood to large muscles in your legs and arms. Your fight-or-flight response then "burns off" those calories. The problem is this: Most often you don't have the option to fight or flee, yet your body is still releasing catecholamines that it doesn't use up. And your heart rate and blood pressure, as well as your stress level, remain elevated. The best way to get rid of those chemicals? Simulate the fight or flight: Walk or run.

11. You'll Have a Healthier Heart. Exercise helps to clear the fats that contribute to disease by stimulating fat-clearing enzymes. Fats are either broken down and excreted or taken up by muscle and fat tissue. Either way, they're out of the bloodstream and less able to increase LDL cholesterol and heart disease risks. This also raises levels of HDL, which protects against heart disease. When a heart is well conditioned, it is like any other muscle. It becomes stronger and more efficient. A normal heart beats at a rate of approximately seventy beats per minute at rest or about 100,000 beats a day. The well-conditioned heart can actually beat as few as forty times a minute at rest or approximately 50,000 beats per day. A well-conditioned heart conserves energy and can supply oxygen-rich blood to the rest of the body with half the effort.

12. You'll Be a More Creative Thinker. According to many recent studies, regular aerobic exercise can improve your memory, enhance your imagination, and make you more creative. The right side of your brain—the area that specializes in creative thought and solving problems—becomes more active when you exercise. It ignites your ability to solve problems, thrive under pressure, and perform at peak levels of effectiveness. As you dramatically increase your oxygen uptake, as well as the production of the red corpuscles that carry oxygen to your brain, the influx enhances the functioning of every organ in your body. Your thinking power receives a forceful boost because 25 percent of your blood is in your brain at any time during exercise.

13. You'll Protect Against Serious Disease. A Harvard University study found that women who run regularly produce a less potent form of estrogen than women who don't, resulting in half the risk of developing breast cancer. Researchers at the Harvard School of Public Health found that a thirty-minute brisk walk or jog cut the risk of colon cancer in half. And physicians at Case Western Reserve University and University Hospitals of Cleveland report that regular exercise seems to reduce the risk of developing Alzheimer's disease. Exercise enhances your immune system, and generally improves the function of almost every organ and system in your body. One study found that people who walked briskly for forty-five minutes a day, five times a week, had half as many colds and flus as nonexercisers.

14. You'll Handle Stress Better. Regular exercise can also help protect against the physical effects of daily stress, according to a report in the November 1999 issue of the *Annals of Behavioral Medicine*. In the study, college students who exercised on a regular basis were more likely to take life's daily stresses in stride, compared with their less physically active counterparts. Previous studies have shown that mental stress takes a toll on physical health, causing such problems as increases in blood sugar levels among diabetics, worsening of joint pain in people with arthritis, and symptoms of psychological distress such as anxiety and depression. Minor, everyday stress contributes to the development and exacerbation of physical and mental health problems. However, people experiencing minor stress develop different degrees of symptoms, depending on their level of physical activity. During periods of high stress, those who reported exercising less frequently had 37 percent more physical symptoms than their counterparts who exercised more often. In addition, highly stressed students who did less exercise reported 21 percent more anxiety than those who exercised more frequently. Exercise helps people get their mind off stressors. This temporary escape from the pressure of stressors acts as a kind of rejuvenation process.

Get F.I.T.T.

You don't have to take up the latest exercise craze to become fit. You can forge your own path, at your own pace, and in your own direction. The frequency, intensity, and duration of your workouts will influence the extent of the health benefits you reap. The type and time of exercise you choose will determine whether you stick with it.

Consider this exercise guide to be F.I.T.T.:

Frequency—Four to six days a week. Exercising less will produce some benefit, but not enough. Exercising more may be useful for athletic training, but can lead to injury.

Intensity—At a level where you feel slightly out of breath, without gasping. Exercise should not hurt. If something hurts, stop and rest. If the pain persists, check with your doctor.

Time—Thirty to sixty minutes, at a time of day when you feel good and your schedule allows you to build a routine.

Type—Whatever type of aerobic exercise you enjoy (or could enjoy) and can do regularly.

Choose a time of day that best suits your schedule. Is it early morning? This is a great choice to beat schedule surprises later in the day. Research has shown that those who begin exercising in the morning are more likely to be at it a year later. Another reason to set the alarm for morning exercise is that after a night's fast, two-thirds of the calories you burn come from stored fat rather than stored glycogen.

If you do exercise first thing, grab a glass of energy-boosting juice

LOSE TWICE AS MANY POUNDS

Researchers at the University of Pittsburgh School of Medicine found that women who exercised for at least 150 minutes a week (that's 30 minutes, five times a week) lost nearly twice as many pounds—25 versus 14—as women who exercised less. Losing weight and keeping it off may require more exercise than previously thought—maybe as much as an hour each day, according to this new research.

In another study from Brown University, researchers found that 2,500 people who lost an average of 60 pounds and kept it off for a year exercised about an hour a day. Most of the people in this study walked about 10 miles a week, then did aerobics, weight lifting, or other activities.

A key to remember is that the more fit you are, the more efficiently you'll burn the calories you eat. If three people of similar weight exercise for 50 minutes at a moderately high intensity, the least fit person would burn about 250 calories, the moderately fit person about 400 calories, and the very fit person about 600 calories.

first (4 to 6 ounces of apple, white grape, or unsweetened cranberry juice is great), then eat breakfast right after your workout. If you exercise outside, pay attention to the weather. If you live in a hot climate, be sure you are drinking lots and lots of water to replenish the fluids you are losing to perspiration. And don't forget your water needs even when it's very cold outside. You can still exercise in winter, but be sure to bundle up in layered clothing that can "wick" the perspiration away from your skin. And cover your head and hands.

If you choose midday as your exercise time, don't let it interfere with your lunchtime fueling or let the exercise break turn your lunch break into a frenzied spin. If you don't have at least an hour, exercise will best wait for another time of day.

If you combine lunch and a workout, be sure you have your midmorning power snack about two hours before your midday workout, then have a piece of fruit (a quick-release carbohydrate) and a 12-ounce glass of water right before you warm up. Exercise for thirty minutes, freshen up, and then have at least a fifteen-minute lunch.

Is early evening best for you? Although this is a difficult time to stay consistent (easy to "just say no" after a hectic day), it's a tremendous time to take advantage of the stress-busting, energizing power of exercise. By diverting yourself from your day's activities, you can downshift from stress to relaxation. It's a good time also to review the day's events—the good, the bad, and the ugly—and get a read on how you feel about them.

If you exercise after dinner, make it a half-hour afterward so you won't be doing battle with your natural digestion process. And don't exercise within half an hour of bedtime; your geared-up metabolism can interfere with restful sleep.

Aerobic workouts are best for morning and midday, serving to maximize energy, reduce tension, and enhance physical and mental performance. Cross-training and interval training (more about these later) can energize your performance even more. Anaerobic work,

25 WAYS TO BURN 250 CALORIES

Activity	Minutes to burn 250 calories
Cleaning the House	68
Cooking	93
Dancing	58
Doing Laundry	64
Gardening	56
Golfing	50
Hiking	52
Ironing	132
In-Line Skating	36
Jumping Rope	26
Making Love	36
Mowing the Lawn	38
Playing Frisbee	43
Playing the Piano	104
Playing Racquetball	24
Playing Tag with Kids	29
Playing Tennis	39
Playing Volleyball	83
Scrubbing Floors	39
Shopping	81
Surfing the Net	148
Swimming	27
Vacuuming	66
Walking the Dog	54
Walking Fast	44

such as conditioning and strength training, may tire you out and is best saved for later in the day.

Household Aerobics

No time to get to the gym because of all those household chores? Just get busy and get them done—and you'll get a fitness reward in the process. Studies have shown that you can ward off weight gain, lower blood pressure, and improve your cholesterol levels just by adding even a little extra activity to your day, instead of a full-fledged workout. Research done at the Cooper Center for Aerobics Research in Dallas shows that to improve your fitness you have to get your heart rate up, but that can be done if you just get moving.

The ways to increase your level of activity without having to adopt a program or invest chunks of time—or money—are endless. And, over time, being more active during the day can have a significant effect on weight loss and maintenance. And bear in mind that the harder you work, the more calories you'll burn. By pushing yourself to walk faster, scrub harder, or dance more vigorously, you can burn as many as 40 percent more calories in the same amount of time.

The point is that *any* amount of physical activity can improve your level of fitness. Fitness is not thinness or being bulked up—it is being able to perform demanding activities without getting out of breath or becoming unduly fatigued.

No Pain, No Gain?

If you don't like exercising for the sake of exercise, just do fun things to make you active: Take the dog out for a walk, chase a football with the neighborhood kids, get your toddler out for a power stroll, jog, swim, bike, dance. Even gardening and mowing the lawn counts. Or find a passion: ballroom dancing, tennis, volleyball, hiking. If you love it, you'll do it.

The notion of "no pain, no gain" is an exercise lie. If you are in pain, you'll stop exercising or get hurt, and the benefits of activity will come screeching to a halt. The key with exercise is not to let it become a stress. Too much, too hard—two to three hours of hammering the body—zaps energy. Moderation in all things, even exercise, are the age-old words of wisdom.

Before beginning or increasing physical activity, take some precautions to ensure a healthy start. To avoid soreness and injury, start out slowly and gradually build up to the desired amount to give your body time to adjust. Most healthy individuals can do this safely.

But if you have chronic health problems such as heart disease, diabetes, asthma, or obesity, you should consult your doctor before you increase your level of physical activity. Also, the American College of Sports Medicine recommends that healthy women over fifty and men over forty who wish to start a vigorous exercise program should check with their doctor to make sure they do not have risk factors for heart disease or any other health problem. Women under fifty and men under forty should also see a physician if they have two or more risk factors for heart disease, such as elevated blood pressure or cholesterol levels, smoking, diabetes, or obesity. And at any age, you should check with your physician first if you have cardiovascular, lung, or joint or muscular disorders (or symptoms that suggest such disorders).

At the very least, you may want to get a fitness physical, which can be performed by your doctor or wellness professional, before you start exercising. An ideal fitness physical is an "all-points check" that tests the following: cholesterol level, heart stress response (an electrocardiogram or "EKG"), lung capacity (in a "VO2 max" challenge), fat-to-lean body composition, blood pressure, and resting heart rate. This battery of tests helps you to discover if there are any potential risk factors in your planned exercise program, and to set realistic goals. It's a terrific benchmark, and can be highly motivating.

A Well-Rounded Workout

Fitness is most easily understood by examining its components. Basically, four types of exercise are needed to provide the best workout and to work all the muscles of your body: warm-up/cool down, aerobic exercise, conditioning/strength exercise, and stretching for flexibility.

Warming Up/Cooling Down

Use warm-up exercises, such as light side-to-side movements, to limber up your muscles and prevent injuries from the other types of exercise. Never skip the warm-up. Muscles work best when they're warmer than normal body temperature, and the warm-up prepares your muscles for the workout. A warm-up also allows your oxygen supply to get ready for what is to come, alerting your body to oncoming shock or stress.

You can warm up with stretching, jumping jacks, skipping rope, or jogging in place. You can also warm up with stretching and then beginning a less intense version of your exercise activity—for example, walking before jogging. An adequate warm-up time is three to five minutes.

Then, at the end of your exercise time, spend three to five minutes cooling down. This allows your body's cardiovascular system to return to normal gradually, preferably over a ten- to fifteen-minute period. This can be considered a "warm-up in reverse" because it consists of the same types of exercises as your warm-up.

The warm-up and the cool-down are just as important as the main event. Both can prevent many of the common injuries that take you out of the race.

Aerobic Exercise

Aerobic exercise is any large-muscle activity that gets your heart pumping and that you can sustain for twenty to sixty minutes. Jumping rope, jogging, cycling, stepping, and other cardiovascular activities are aerobic exercises that leave you energized.

Your heart and lungs work together to supply oxygen to tissues in your body. Aerobic exercise forces the lungs and heart to work harder and, in so doing, strengthens and conditions them. It is crucial for overall body wellness and for fanning the flame of the metabolic fire that burns fat. Continuous activity most activates the metabolism, not the stop-stand-start activity of softball, volleyball, or golf. And the routine of exercise is what builds a conditioned body, one that adapts much more resiliently to stress.

The minute you start to exercise, your metabolic rate (the amount of energy you expend) increases to somewhere between five and twenty times what you expend sitting down. This change is very healthy when done on a regular basis. The goal is to try for some kind of activity every day. Even if it's not a hard workout at the gym, just a walk after dinner can do miraculous things for your body.

Vary your routine to rev up the calorie burn. Different forms of exercise build and strengthen muscles in more parts of the body. Cross-training is a technique you can employ that drives up the effectiveness of your aerobic workouts. Quite simply, it is alternating the aerobic activities you do. Instead of using a treadmill four days a week, alternate it with two days of biking. Instead of running every

EXERCISE BEFORE YOU INDULGE

Take a long, brisk walk before your friend's wedding, and the hors d'oeuvres and cake may not be a heart attack on your plate. In addition to its benefits to your waistline, exercise can help override some of the nasty effects of fat in your blood.

High-calorie meals cause spikes in the amount of triglycerides in the bloodstream, which wreak havoc on cholesterol by decreasing good HDL and increasing bad LDL. Over time, these contribute to atherosclerosis and heart disease. But researchers recently found that the timing of exercise can affect these fat levels significantly.

When a group of twenty-one men exercised twelve hours before a high-fat meal, they cut the amount of fat in their blood by half. (Exercising one hour before the meal lowered fat by nearly 40 percent.) Working out after a high-fat meal reduced it by only 5 percent.

day, run three times a week, swim for two, and cycle for another. Your body perceives the different forms of exercise as more demanding (even though they may seem less demanding), and will trigger greater internal exertion. As a result, you will burn more fat for fuel and become a more efficient energy producer.

Interval training is a technique in which you vary the intensity at which you exercise. If you normally jog at a slow pace, periodically pick up the pace to a run, maybe for a minute, and then return to a slow jog. Alternate this during your entire exercise time. It can give a significant boost to your fitness gains and energy levels.

If your main concern is shedding some body fat, the key is to do longer, more frequent aerobic sessions at an easier pace. This approach burns more calories. Even though vigorous exercise burns more calories per minute than an easy effort, an extra fifteen or thirty minutes of easy exercise will more than make up the difference.

Longer bouts of exercise also burn proportionally more fat. Harder but shorter exercise draws more on carbohydrates. If you walk or do some other activity for more than an hour, your body will start to burn significantly more fat for the rest of the workout. Why? Because the carbohydrate stores in your muscles begin running low after an hour.

Once you've settled into a routine of exercise:
- Do five to seven aerobic workouts a week.
- Make your effort as easy as possible so that you're able to exercise continuously for forty-five to sixty minutes without strain.
- Try to do one or more "long" workouts (over an hour) per week.
- Ignore any pounds lost in the first week (which are mostly water) and concentrate on a steady, consistent weight reduction of about a half-pound to one pound per week.

Conditioning/Strength Exercises

Conditioning or strength exercises are those that tone, shape, and define the muscles through repetitive movements against resistance. Conditioning exercises activate the metabolism by making demands on the muscles that change their chemistry, making them more energy efficient. Conditioning increases muscle strength and mass by putting more than the usual amount of strain on a muscle that stimulates the growth of small force-generating proteins inside each muscle cell. These proteins feed the "fibers" that grow during exercise. When you make muscles work harder, you actually tear these fibers. As they rebuild, they get stronger and bigger, resulting in harder, tighter, and more defined muscles.

Resistance training can also have a beneficial effect on your body composition. As sedentary people age, from about age twenty or so, they lose 1 percent of their muscle mass each year. By age forty, it has amounted to 20 percent. Between the ages of twenty and sixty, inactive people can lose up to 40 percent of their muscle mass. And the flabbier muscles are, the less muscle fuel (energy) they can store. That means less strength and stamina for you. By the age of forty, up to one-half pound of muscle—and the energy stocked inside—is generally replaced with a half-pound of fat.

By reversing this process, weight training can see you into middle age with the energy, strength, and metabolism you had at twenty. As your muscles grow and become more active, the level of energy within the muscles increases, making you more vital. In addition, stronger muscles offer more support to your joints, pump up your sports performance, improve your balance, and help prevent injuries. And regular weight training exercises can boost your cardiovascular health by improving your levels of good cholesterol (HDL). Resistance training also strengthens your bones and helps increase bone mineral mass to help prevent osteoporosis, a disease that afflicts twenty million women in the United States.

A conditioning or resistance workout usually involves various exercises that focus on different muscle groups. This is the essence of circuit training on machines like Nautilus, which were built for this purpose. Normally the exerciser does one to three "sets" of each exercise (a set can be anywhere from eight to fifteen repetitions, and takes about one minute to complete). A typical session lasts about thirty minutes. But any kind of repetitive resistance training is effective, whether it's circuit training on weight machines; an arm workout with barbells or full soup cans; calisthenics such as chin-ups, push-ups, and sit-ups; or arm and leg extensions with exercise bands.

Just doing a few simple ten- to fifteen-minute strength-training routines at home or at the gym, two times a week, can turn the tide on muscle loss and activate your metabolism. You may notice an increase in the strength and the size of the exercised muscles in just a few weeks.

The good news is that strength and conditioning exercises are easy! And you don't need to spend a fortune on expensive equipment. A few years ago, I made a $20 investment in a pair of three- to five-pound dumbbells and a rubber exercise band, which is about four inches wide and three feet long and comes in different resistance levels. My best way to build strength has been to lift weights in three sets of eight to twelve repetitions. Lifting a lighter weight for more repetitions is the technique I use to build endurance and tone.

Here are some other tips to keep in mind as you build conditioning into your workout:

- If you plan to work out at home, purchase a pair of three- to five-pound hand-held weights or adjustable-weight dumbbells (with metal plates that can be added or taken off).
- Before trying any strength exercise, practice it several times with a very light weight, to learn the movement correctly.
- If you have access to a gym or health club that has Nautilus machines or other weight-lifting machines, sign up for an orientation to learn the proper use of each machine. You may consider a session with a certified personal trainer to get an individualized program worked out for you to reach your goals.
- Start with weights that feel comfortable for you and that allow you to do eight to twelve repetitions without pain. If you can't make eight repetitions of a given exercise, switch to a lower weight. Each lifting motion should take two seconds (counting "*one*, one thousand; *two*, one thousand"), while the recovery motion (returning to starting position) should take four seconds. If you're using dumbbells, two sets (with a couple of minutes of rest in between) are recommended. If you're using a weight machine, one set per exercise is enough.
- As you work out for several weeks or months, your muscles will get noticeably stronger, to the point where you'll need to increase the amount of weight you're lifting to continue improving. Whenever the twelfth repetition becomes easy on a given exercise, add three to five pounds to each dumbbell, or ten pounds to the load on the weight machine for that exercise.
- Each strength workout should include a variety of exercises that work both the pushing and pulling muscles of the upper body (arms, shoulders, abdomen, and back) and lower body (legs,

hips, and buttocks).

- Always allow at least forty-eight hours of recovery time between strength workouts, to give your muscle tissue time to rebuild.
- Choose your equipment wisely. For example, vinyl-coated dumbbells are comfortable to lift, and the bright colors lift your spirits, too. These are great weights for beginners because they come in one-pound increments (up to eight pounds), with a ten-pound option as you progress. (Beyond ten pounds, you'll have to opt for the more traditional chrome or cast-iron types.) Hand weights are also a good option for beginners, especially for people who have arthritis in their hands. Designed with either a strap or handle, you don't have to use a tight grip to hold onto them. Strapping weights to your ankles or wrists instead of carrying them in the hands is another great choice for people with arthritis, high blood pressure, or any other condition in which you should avoid tight grips. And whether you exercise at home or travel a lot, elastic exercise bands are a great way to enhance your workout. These bands are lightweight, easy to use, and allow you to do exercises that normally require expensive machines.

The Exercises

These are some exercises that can form the core of a regular strength-training program. You may want to begin with the first four exercises below and supplement them with the next four exercises if and when you want to expand your strength training program.

Weight Training

DUMBBELL SQUAT (LOWER BODY) OR LEG EXTENSION MACHINE

Stand holding a dumbbell in each hand with your feet flat on the floor, shoulder-width apart, and your arms down at your sides. Keeping your head up and your back straight, slowly lower your hips until your thighs are parallel with the floor. Then return slowly to starting position, still keeping head up and back straight. Repeat eight to twelve times.

Dumbbell Lunge (lower body) or Leg Curl machine

Stand holding a dumbbell in each hand, with your arms down at your sides and your feet slightly less than shoulder-width apart. Looking directly ahead and keeping your left leg straight, take a long step forward with your right leg, bending your right knee so that the knee is lined up directly above your right ankle. Distributing your weight equally on both legs, bend your back leg until your knee is almost touching the ground. Then push slowly off your right foot, stepping back into your starting position. Repeat eight to twelve times, then switch legs and repeat.

Dumbbell Chest Press (upper body) or Chest Press machine

Lie face up on a flat bench or on the floor, with your feet flat on the floor, and hold a dumbbell in each hand. Extend your arms and then lower them to starting position against your chest (your elbows should point out to either side). Slowly push the dumbbells upward together until your arms are fully extended and the dumbbells are directly above your chest. Repeat eight to twelve times.

Dumbbell Row (upper body) or Lateral Pull-Down machine

Holding a dumbbell in your right hand, rest your left knee on a low bench or step, and place your left (free) hand down flat in front of your knee on the same bench. You should be leaning forward so that your back is horizontal, and your right foot should be flat on the floor, with the right knee slightly bent. Lower the dumbbell so that your right arm is fully extended and slowly pull it to your chest, then return slowly to starting position. Do eight to twelve repetitions, then switch sides and repeat.

Dumbbell Curl (upper body) or Biceps machine

Holding a dumbbell in each hand, stand comfortably with your arms down at your sides. Slowly bend your arms, curling both dumbbells up to your shoulders, then slowly return to starting position. Keep your head up and your eyes looking straight ahead at all times.

Dumbbell Triceps Extension (upper body) or Triceps machine

Holding a dumbbell in your right hand, place your left knee on a low bench or chair, and place your left hand in front of it, flat on the bench. Hold the dumbbell with your palm facing inward, and your right elbow slightly bent so the weight is at hip level. Keeping your right shoulder still, slowly straighten your right arm, then slowly return to starting position. Repeat eight to twelve times, then switch arms and repeat.

Dumbbell Shoulder Press (upper body) or Overhead Press machine

Holding a dumbbell in each hand, sit on a bench or a chair with your feet flat on the floor. Position both dumbbells at shoulder level, with your elbows pointing downward. Then slowly press both dumbbells upward, until your arms are straight but not locked (think of squeezing your shoulder blades together as you lift). Then return slowly to starting position. Repeat eight to twelve times.

Dumbbell Deltoid Raise (upper body) or Lateral Raise machine

Standing comfortably and with a dumbbell in each hand, hold your arms at your sides so that your elbows are bent at right angles, with your palms facing downward. Slowly raise both dumbbells until your upper arms are parallel to the ground. Then slowly lower your arms to starting position. Repeat eight to twelve times.

Here are three sample exercises you can do with exercise bands:
- Keeping your arms parallel to the floor, hold the band in front of your chest (at armpit level) with your hands about six inches apart. Slowly bring your elbows toward your back, as if you were squeezing a pencil with your shoulder blades. Hold for two seconds, then bring your elbows forward again. (If this is too difficult for you, use a band with less resistance; if it's too easy, switch to a band with more resistance.)

- Stand on one end of the band and hold the other in one hand. With your palm facing upward, slowly bring the band up to your shoulder, using only the lower part of your arm. It's important to keep the elbow close to the body and the upper arm straight. Repeat with the other arm.

- To target the large latissimus dorsi muscle of your back, a muscle particularly difficult to get at using dumbbells, attach a band to the top of a door using a specially designed door anchor. (If you don't secure the band, it may slide off the door and smack you in the face!) Then sit or kneel on the floor, facing the door and holding the band so that it and your arms are fully extended. Your hands should be about shoulder-width apart. Squeezing your shoulder blades, pull your hands down toward your chest. Elbows should be pointing behind you and down. Hold, and then release.

Calisthenics to Reduce Belly Bulge

No matter what the cause of extra abdominal fat—a recent baby, too many brews, or too much time on the sofa—this program will work for you. Do these six exercises three or four times a week to tone and tighten your abs. If you're doing these at home, an exercise mat is a wise investment.

Get started today! But go slowly for best results. Forget doing hundreds of crunches. You'll get a flatter tummy quicker if you slow down. Each repetition of an exercise should take about six to eight seconds to complete. For example, slowly count one, two, three, four as you *lift* during a crunch, and then five, six, seven, eight as you *lower*. If you experience back pain with any of these exercises, stop the exercise and check with your doctor before continuing. Do each exercise three or four times a week.

CRUNCH

Lying on a mat or carpeted floor, place your hands lightly behind your head, bend your knees, and put your feet flat on the floor.

Using your abs, slowly lift your head, shoulders, and upper back off the mat. Keep your abs tight and exhale on the way up. Hold, and then lower. Do ten to fifteen repetitions.

TWISTING CRUNCH

Start in the crunch position. As you lift, twist your torso, bringing your left shoulder toward your right knee at the top of the crunch. Hold, and then lower. Repeat on the other side. Do ten to fifteen repetitions on each side.

ROLLDOWN

Sit on the floor with your knees bent, feet flat. Keeping your arms out in front of you, slowly roll down—one vertebrae at a time—until you're lying on the floor. Then roll to your side and sit up. Do four to six repetitions.

LEG DROP

Lying on your back, bend at your knees and hips so your legs form a right angle. Keeping your back pressed to the mat, slowly lower your right leg until your toe touches the mat. Then slowly return it to the starting position. If your back starts to arch, stop at that point. As your abs get stronger, you'll be able to go farther. Do four to six repetitions with each leg and then do both legs together.

SITTING KNEE LIFT

Sit up straight in a firm, armless chair. Place your hands on the sides of the chair in front of your hips. Tightening your abs and supporting yourself with your hands, slowly pull your knees up toward your chest. Hold and then slowly lower. Keep your lower back against the chair back. This is an advanced exercise, so you may want to start by alternating your legs, lifting one at a time. Do four to six repetitions.

As with any other exercise program, before starting a strength-training regimen, you need to get a medical exam to rule out any possible underlying health problems or any existing conditions that could be aggravated.

Exercising for Flexibility

Flexibility is the ability of joints and muscles to achieve a full range of motion. Exercising for flexibility helps prevent injuries, improves your posture, provides for better breathing, and even lowers blood pressure. Despite popular opinion, there's no evidence that you should lose flexibility as you build muscle.

Flexibility exercises use gentle, stretching movements to increase the length of your muscles and the effective range of motion in your joints, allowing you to perform better at daily tasks—from bending over to tie your shoe to lifting a baby out of a car seat to carrying a heavy computer bag. They may consist of a series of specific stretching exercises or be part of a larger exercise program such as aerobics or dance classes.

Because one of the main goals of stretching is to lengthen the connective tissue surrounding your muscle fibers, flexibility exercises should be done after you've already warmed up your muscles with a few minutes of aerobic activity. A typical session involves a minute or two on each stretching exercise. As with aerobics, you can break up your stretching routine into shorter sessions before and after your other workouts.

All stretching movements should be done slowly, to the point where you feel a gentle pleasant tension—not pain—in the muscle being stretched. For an effective stretch, you need to hold the position for fifteen to thirty seconds, then work toward holding all stretches for a full minute. Breathe deeply through your nostrils, concentrating on the muscles you're stretching. Never "bounce" as you hold a stretch, because this will activate your stretch reflex (an automatic, protective contraction). If you feel any pain, stop immediately.

If you regularly stretch your muscles after they're fully warmed up—at the end of an aerobic workout, for example—you can gradually increase their resting length by lengthening the connective tissue that surrounds your muscle fibers. Improving flexibility in this way will make movement easier and more fluid. The more often you stretch, the longer your muscles. For maximum benefits, do a stretching routine several times each week.

Here are some flexibility exercises to add in to your exercise routine. The ideal is two thirty-minute flexibility workouts each week, or ten minutes each day incorporated into your aerobic workout.

HAMSTRING STRETCH

Sit with your right leg extended in front of you, your left leg bent with your left sole resting against your right thigh. Place your right hand on the floor slightly behind you as you slowly reach forward with your left hand. Grasp and flex the toes of your right foot, if you can. Repeat four times, then switch legs.

THE BIG V

Lie on your back with legs straight and stretched out to the sides so that they form a V in the air. Flex your feet so that your toes are pointing toward your body. Place your hands on the inside of each thigh just above the knee and slowly press until you feel a gentle tension in your inner thighs. Repeat four times.

TOWEL STRETCH

Stand with your feet together, knees slightly bent. With your arms overhead, hold a towel taut (if you feel too much tension, get a longer towel so that your hands are positioned farther apart). Take the towel a few inches behind your head, then slowly lower it. Keep your elbows soft. When you feel the stretch across your chest, take a few deep breaths and hold it. As your flexibility improves, slide your hands closer together.

CALF STRETCH

Stand comfortably with your hands on your hips, or place both hands on a wall, shoulder-width apart, and step forward with your right foot (about a half-shoulder's width). Bend both knees, keeping your feet flat on the floor, and shift your weight to your forward foot. Slowly lower your hips, until you feel a gentle stretching sensation in the calf muscle and Achilles tendon of your left (rear) leg. Hold for fifteen to thirty seconds, then switch legs and repeat.

TRICEPS STRETCH

Stand tall, with your feet shoulder-width apart. Reach down the middle of your back with your right hand, pointing your elbow toward the ceiling. Keeping your shoulders down, use your left hand to pull your right elbow gently toward the center of your body. Imagine that you're trying to align your forearm with your spine to form a continuous straight line. Repeat four times. Switch arms.

CROSS-LEGGED PULL

Lie on your back with your right leg bent, foot planted on the floor. Cross your left ankle over your right thigh. Clasp your hands behind your right thigh and gently coax the leg toward your chest. Feel the deep stretch in your left hip. Repeat four times, then switch sides.

Walk for Life

Want to drop a size, stabilize hormones, sleep better, and live longer? I can't say it enough: putting one foot in front of the other does your body, mind, and spirit a world of good!

There are many unquestionably good exercises, but all are not everyone's cup of tea. For those that cringe at the thought of jogging, can't easily get to a pool for swimming, and don't have the time, place, or desire for aerobic dancing, fitness walking is a tremendous alternative.

Walking is structured, simple, easy, quick, and cheap—and is guaranteed to make you feel better and look better in just a couple of weeks. It's also a social contribution: researchers have concluded that you help the national economy just by taking a walk. Two doctors at Brown University have calculated the amount spent nationally each year on heart-disease treatment and the added amount wasted as a result of lost employee productivity. They estimated that $5.6 billion in health care costs would be saved if only one out of ten nonexercising adults started a regular walking program.

Even if you haven't exercised in a long time, remember that walking is natural and easy. You need not "gear up" mentally, so walking is easy to build into your life's routine. Even if you don't walk far, just get out and move.

Six Reasons Why Walking Rules

1. You Can Do It for Life. Forty years from now, you may not be rollerblading every morning, but you could still be walking—around your neighborhood, to the park, maybe in the mall. With little risk of injury and great opportunity to see gains in fitness, walking is a sport you can keep for life.

2. You Can Run or Walk No Matter What Your Body Type. You may not ever have the muscular makeup to do marathons, but as long as you start slowly to prevent injuries, anyone—short, tall, big, or small—can walk or run.

3. You Can Walk No Matter What Your Condition. Whether you're pregnant, elderly, or obese; with arthritis, diabetes or osteoporosis; even recovering from heart surgery or chronic fatigue—you can walk safely.

4. You Can Lose Weight Walking. The faster you walk (and the more you weigh), the more calories you use.

5. You Can Get Well Walking. Walking's health benefits include an increase in HDL levels, a reduced risk of bone loss and resulting fractures, a decrease in blood pressure, a stabilization of blood sugar levels in diabetics, and an increase in mobility for people with arthritis.

6. You Can Feel Well by Walking. Walking has immense emotional benefits. It counters depression, relieves stress, and refreshes your spirit. You can talk to God, yourself, or a walking companion.

Turning a Walk Into a Workout

Find a block of time in the morning (before breakfast) or after work (ideally, before dinner) to go for a brisk walk around your neighborhood. If you are traveling, or don't feel comfortable walking in your own neighborhood, stop off on the way home at an area where you feel safe. Just remember to pack your walking shoes!

Look for a shoe that offers stability, good arch support, and durability, with a maximum half-inch heel height. The heel should be rolled and tapered, and the heel cushion should be about one-half to three-quarters of an inch thick. Combine good shoes with good-quality athletic socks that fit smoothly and evenly on your feet. Don't wear running shoes for walking; walking shoes help your feet roll along in a heel-toe motion and have more flexible soles for faster walking.

Before and after each walk, gently stretch to keep muscle soreness and tightness to a minimum. Do gentle, nonbouncing stretches for your shin muscles, calf muscles and tendons, hamstrings and front thighs with a slow, steady pull until you feel the muscles ache slightly. Trunk rotations (turning the upper body while feet remain planted) and side bends are helpful as well. Hold each stretch for fifteen seconds. Do these stretches even on days you don't exercise, to keep your muscles from tightening.

Walk fast enough to work up a light sweat (swing your arms, take long, but comfortable strides), but not so fast that you become breathless. This is your ideal "aerobic" pace. You should always be able to talk to a companion (or hum to yourself) during exercise. If you can't do this, slow your pace. When you feel like extending yourself a bit more, research indicates that you will benefit as much from extending time as from increasing pace and stepping more frequently rather than trying to stretch your stride, which can injure your knees.

EXERCISING IN THE ZONE

If you're walking for a half hour or more each day, you might want to consider buying a fun little gadget called a pulse meter that can tell you at a glance whether you're getting the most out of your exercise. Worn on the wrist or chest, a pulse meter monitors your heart rate so you can see if you're exercising in your target zone.

What's your target zone? It varies depending on your age. Your maximum heart rate is the fastest your heart can beat. The best activity level is 60 to 75 percent of this maximum rate. In this zone, your muscles are moving, you're breathing deeply, your blood is delivering ample amounts of oxygen to your body systems, and you're burning fat as your major fuel source. At this level, you should be breathing deeply but comfortably enough that you can hold a conversation or sing to yourself.

To find your heart rate target zone, subtract your age from 220. Your exercise zone will be 60 to 75 percent of that number. So, a forty-five-year-old would subtract forty-five from 220, getting an average maximum heart rate (100 percent) of 175. Sixty to 75 percent of this number would be 105 to 131 beats per minute.

When you begin your exercise program, aim for the lower part of your heart rate target zone (60 percent) during the first few months. As you get into better shape, gradually build up to the higher part of your target zone (75 percent).

Proper posture is very important to protect against fatigue and injuries. Stand up straight and walk with your ears, shoulders, hips, knees, and ankles in a vertical line. Keep your head erect, chin pulled in toward your neck, back straight, and buttocks and stomach tucked in. Avoid leaning forward when walking to prevent back strain.

Walking will satisfy all your body's needs for aerobic exercise if you do it in such a way as to raise your heart rate to its training zone. If your heart rate is not elevated at the end of a forty-five minute walk, try walking faster, at least part of the time, or look for some long, gradual hills to climb. You may also try walking with weights.

Plan to get some walking in every day, or at least four to five days a week. In a few weeks, your exercise program will be a habit and you'll feel uncomfortable if you have to miss a day. I've done a lot of different forms of exercise at different times in my life, but I always come back to walking. It's simply the best exercise for me to rely on to keep my body operating at its metabolic best.

Sticking With It

Just knowing the benefits of exercise isn't enough; more people don't exercise than do. What's the problem? For a lot of us, it's just that exercise is no fun—and it's hard to stick with something every day that's not. The only way it will become part of your daily life is if you find an exercise that matches your lifestyle, your fitness needs, and your own definition of enjoyment. Follow these guidelines to increase your enjoyment of an exercise routine.

Know Yourself

The exercises you'll find most enjoyable will probably be those you feel you can best handle. If you have difficulty with eye-hand coordination, you may be frustrated by a sport like tennis but would do well with walking or swimming. If you are not naturally flexible, you may be happier with bicycling than ballet. And you may just want to choose aerobic gardening! Exercise doesn't have to be running a marathon—you just need to get moving, and do it consistently. Playing with your kids or grandchildren may work just fine!

Consider Your Current Condition

If you are overweight, choosing an activity that involves pounding on your feet, such as running or aerobic dance, may stress your joints by placing too much weight on them. Try riding a stationary bike or swimming instead. And remember, if you're over thirty-five, see a health professional for an "all-points" check before beginning an exercise program.

Use the Buddy System

Exercising with a friend will not only give you an opportunity to socialize, but you'll also be more motivated to show up and keep your commitment. Other people's enthusiasm and energy may be just the inspiration you need.

Distract Yourself

If your exercise of choice isn't particularly interesting, combine it with something that is. Do the StairMaster while listening to books on tape, or sing along to uplifting music while walking on the treadmill.

Have Fun

Take up a sport that allows you to get exercise while working on skills and having fun. Volleyball, racquetball, in-line skating, even badminton are activities that provide terrific fitness benefits but don't feel like exercise. Pick activities that reduce stress, not those that add to it. If risk-taking isn't your idea of fun, leave skydiving to someone else!

Remember the Payoff

Keep your focus on how good you'll feel after you exercise. Keep envisioning exercise as a sword that cuts away at the stress response. Remind yourself of the long-term benefits you're getting: better energy, a better body, and better health. Choosing to exercise daily is giving yourself a precious gift. And your body was created to reward you by strengthening your "armor": building up protective barriers against heart disease, diabetes, bone loss, arthritis, even cancer.

Fine-Tune Your Workout

You're thinking of chucking it all because you're not seeing the payoff? You're still carrying around an extra fifteen pounds? Or maybe you're not getting stronger, faster, or any more energized? Before you give up, use these five steps to fine-tune your workouts for maximum results:

1. Be a Little Pushy. If you've been doing the same type of exercise for more than three months, you may be stuck. It's easy to amble on walks or coast along on your bike. But for meaningful results, you've got to challenge yourself. Push to go just a little faster, a little longer (even an extra five minutes can do the trick), or to do it more often. To avoid injury, though, increase only one aspect of your workout at a time.

2. Experiment. The more proficient your muscles become at a particular activity, the fewer calories you burn. Add a new activity such as biking, swimming, jump-roping, even kickboxing or volleyball to your usual exercise routine. You'll burn more calories as you master a new skill—and you'll have fun! Cross-training is also a great way to prevent injuries and boredom.

3. Be Active All Day. Don't think that you can veg out the rest of the day just because you took a low-impact aerobics class or a brisk, hour-long walk. The 300 to 400 calories that you likely burned won't make up for all the calories you're not burning throughout the day thanks to the TV remote, automatic garage-door opener, e-mail, and even the electric can-opener. It's estimated that in the past twenty-five years, labor-saving devices have decreased the number of calories we burn daily by 800 or more.

4. Check Your Fridge. Exercise is key to losing weight and keeping it off, but you can't ignore what you eat. An extra slice of pizza, for example, can put right back the 240 calories you burned jogging for half an hour. And even if you're choosing low-fat, nutritious foods, eating too much of them can have the same effect. Be aware of what and how much you're eating so that you don't negate the calorie-burning benefits of exercise.

5. Take a Break. Doing too much, particularly vigorous, high-intensity exercise, can actually hinder your progress. Your body needs time to recover from intense workouts in order to get stronger. Take at least two or three days off between these high-intensity workouts to let your muscles recover, or mix in some lower-intensity walking, swimming, or stretching.

If you are ready to move beyond the reasons not to exercise and join the ranks of those who successfully develop a regular exercise routine and enjoy its benefits, take note: Initiating a well-designed exercise plan will create a wave of positive changes in your life. You'll work with a higher level of energy, think with greater mental clarity and concentration, build confidence, quell negative anxiety, and cut away at the stress response—and all the while lose body fat; build and tone firm, lean muscle; stabilize blood chemistry; and increase your strength. It's an incredible package that shouldn't be hard to sell, even to ourselves!

Exercise is a powerful tool in your pound-shedding and stress-fighting tool chest. Another is healthy, full breaths of air—and lots and lots of water.

CHAPTER 5

S

M

AIR AND WATER

R

T

The Air Out There

Ever breathe a sigh of relief? Gasp in shock or pain? Feel the need to vent at someone? These all express the close connection between the way we breathe and how we feel.

The pressure of a deadline can leave us wiped out for the afternoon. Fear makes us tense our muscles, which leads to fatigue, just as if we were working out. Fear can also make us hold our breath, depriving us of oxygen. This not only can lead to fatigue, but it can kick up the stress response and slam shut the fat cell door.

Breathing isn't something we normally have to think about—we inhale and exhale at a fairly steady pace, without much thought or worry over how we're doing. We take on average 28,000 breaths each day. But how we take those breaths contributes to our body's metabolic response—it revs it up or locks it down. While losing weight, we have much to gain from learning how to breathe correctly.

In addition, deep and slow oxygenating breaths are one of the simplest things you can do to relieve stress, energize yourself, and keep control of yourself in any situation. Healthy breathing can help you overcome the low energy and high stress levels that result from rapid, shallow, or deep, heaving breaths.

Again, because breathing seems so simple, so automatic, it's difficult to think that our metabolism and energy can be boosted just from taking a breath of air. And it certainly is automatic, but so is eating. And how many people do that right?

Back to Basics

Getting the right amount of oxygen into the bloodstream depends on a balance of carbon dioxide and oxygen in the blood. When you breathe in a panicked way, each breath throws that balance off. But you can actually train yourself to breathe in a way that energizes you.

When you're relaxed, you breathe slowly and deeply, inhaling vital, energy-producing oxygen. When you're tense or just not breathing correctly, you tend to breathe lightly and rapidly from your chest, which delivers less oxygen to your body's cells. As professional singers will tell you, only 30 percent of your full oxygen capacity is available when you're not breathing in a deep, diaphragmatic way— it suffocates your blood cells.

To test your breathing, place one hand on your upper chest and one hand on your abdomen. If the hand on your chest rises when you inhale and contracts when you exhale, you're chest breathing. This type of breathing brings in large amounts of air at one time and activates the fight-or-flight alarm reaction. This is good in a life-threatening emergency, but not in daily living.

Chest breathing keeps your body in a state of chronic stress. It also impairs circulation, depletes energy, and slows the metabolism because without adequate oxygen the body cells cannot burn fat effectively nor produce a full measure of energy. The brain reads this as stress, and produces stress hormones. Yet the shallow breathing that accompanies stress decreases the oxygen intake and transfer, and we become even more stressed. Another vicious cycle.

Studies suggest that 80 percent of us don't know how to breathe in a metabolically activating and energizing way; we put our emphasis on inhalation, but the energy and stress release is in exhalation.

Freeze for a moment, holding your body in its exact position. Notice that your shoulders may be shrugged or tense. Correct your posture; imagine being suspended from above with your head erect, light and alert. Next, exhale slowly, draining your lungs—concentrating on the stress being blown out of your body, out through the mouth. Now, slowly fill your chest with air, taking the air in through your nostrils. Expand your diaphragm (the cone-shaped muscle that forms the floor of your chest cavity) by pushing your stomach down and out. Then breathe again...in and out...fully. In and out...in and out.

Release and Relax

Breathing in this way—from your diaphragm—tells your body: "Everything is okay...you're in control." So, before the pressures of life attack again, take two minutes to practice this type of breath work.

The best way to get started in a focused releasing/relaxing breath pattern is to place one hand on your upper stomach, just below your chest. Inhale while you imagine you're filling a small balloon inside. Fill it in all directions—top, bottom, forward, backward. Breathe in until you feel comfortably full, but not too full. Your stomach should gently rise and then fall as you exhale. Make the exhalation a little bit longer than you think you should. Hold it for a half-second before you inhale again. Your upper chest should stay flat throughout. Once you're breathing from the right spot, focus on making your breath even and steady. You'll find that your tension dissipates.

Ready to blow a gasket because your computer just froze again? Put your hands flat on your desk and take about fifteen slow, deep breaths. Breathe in, breathe out. You'll feel calmer, and you'll unwind all the energy-depleting tension before it has a chance to overtake you. Practice this energizing and relaxing deep breathing so that you can do it automatically when under stress. Try it whenever the tension builds—in meetings, during a crisis, when you feel tired, unfocused, confused, mad, scared, anxious, or bored.

Repeat breathing "in and out" fully, at least ten times, whenever you feel tired or stressed. Your body and mind will soon feel the release and refreshment.

Overcoming Hyperventilation

Many people are being robbed of energy and metabolic power because they breathe shallowly and rapidly (more than eighteen times per minute), leading to an excessive loss of carbon dioxide. The loss of carbon dioxide due to this chronic hyperventilation affects the blood's hemoglobin, making it less able to carry oxygen throughout the body. So even though you are breathing quickly, you are getting less air. Among the symptoms are fatigue, anxiety, frequent sighing or yawning, and a tingling, coldness, or numbness in the fingers. Many of these symptoms are because you are holding your breath to make up for the carbon dioxide lost in hyperventilating. In addition, you have to work harder to breathe, which in and of itself is tiring.

How to overcome hyperventilation problems? First, sit or stand up straight—correct your posture. Keeping your tummy firmly tucked in when you stand or sit up straight will relax your diaphragm muscles and improve their movement during breathing. Second, if you breathe from your nose, keep your mouth closed. Your nasal passages are too narrow to allow for hyperventilation. Third, practice breathing into a closed paper bag held tightly against your face. With this bag-breathing, carbon dioxide is trapped into the bag, where it is recirculated, preventing carbon dioxide levels from falling. Finally, learn the art of breathing to release stress—getting your breath working for you, not against you.

Learning to Exhale

You can further expand your stress-busting expertise by learning how to manipulate the way you exhale. Because exhaling slows the pulse, a technique called two/one breathing, in which you exhale for twice as long as you inhale, makes diaphragmatic breathing even more effective.

To practice the two/one breathing technique, follow these steps:

1. Sit quietly and do diaphragmatic breathing.
2. When your breathing becomes balanced and even (it will take a few minutes), gently slow your rate of exhalation until you are breathing out for about twice as long as you breathe in. The easiest technique: count six when you exhale, three when you inhale, or eight and four. You shouldn't end up doing deep breathing; you want to alter the rhythmic motion of your lungs, not fill or empty them completely.
3. Once you've established your rhythm of breathing, stop the mental counting and focus on the smoothness and evenness of your breath flow.

You receive more than air through proper breathing—you invite regeneration into your body. Breathing for energy gives you a recharge, along with a sense of rest and relaxation. So take a nice, long, slow breath. Now, take another one. Feel better?

Making Scents

Now, consider the air you are breathing in: Is it pure and clear? Toxic air depresses your immune system—and slows your body. Even the scent in the air can lessen your body's ability to lose weight because of the air quality's effect on your brain chemistry.

Pleasant scents stimulate a nerve in the body that triggers wakefulness and alertness. They also can impact the nerve response that triggers appetite—and satiety.

You don't need fancy fragrances or potpourris—they sometimes overwhelm the olfactory sensors, particularly when synthetic. Go the most natural way you can: Keep a basket of oranges or lemons on your desk, and slice one when you're feeling fatigued. The sniff will trigger alertness. A mint plant on your desk will provide the same boost when you break off a leaf to breathe in its aroma. Because of intriguing research, many Japanese corporations pipe the scent of peppermint through their air-conditioning systems in midafternoon to perk up energy and boost concentration and productivity.

Another energizing scent is jasmine, which actually alters brain waves and energy levels. It increases the beta waves in the frontal lobe of the brain, stimulating alertness. Jasmine plants or essential oils will supply the refreshment.

A splitting headache, and still more to do on the report? Well, a green apple a day may keep your migraine away—smelling it, that is! Research by Dr. Alan Hirsch of the Smell and Taste Treatment and Research Foundation in Chicago found that for those who like the smell of green apples, the scent produces a marked reduction in the severity of their headaches. This may also be related to the alteration of brain waves.

Feeling overwhelmed by the stress of the day? The scent of lavender has been found to induce alpha waves in the back of the brain that relax and calm. Certain scents, such as strawberries and popcorn, can even distract you from the stress you are feeling.

The easiest way to provide the specific scent you need is to purchase a small vial of an essential oil, a concentrated mixture extracted from a plant. (Be sure to get pure, natural scents only, available from natural foods stores, bath and body shops, and certain drug stores.) An effective way to put the scent where it counts is with a small atomizer (less than a dollar) filled with water and just a few drops of the essential oil. Shake before using, then lightly spray on the pulse points of your wrists, or into the air as a freshener.

Some of the more stimulating scents are lemon, peppermint or spearmint, pine, rosemary, eucalyptus, jasmine, and basil. Among the known relaxing scents are lavender, chamomile, orange blossom, rose, marjoram, sage, and patchouli.

The Purifying Power of Plants

Plants give off low levels of hundreds of different chemicals that purify the air. Although the chemicals are designed to protect the plant against insects, they also energize us by protecting against "sick-building syndrome." In addition, plants absorb many toxins like formaldehyde and benzene; the root systems of plants actually feed off pollutants and toxins in the air. After absorbing the contaminants, the plants "breathe back" clean air.

The build-up of air contaminants in many buildings and homes can cause flu-like symptoms and fatigue, even cancer. Plants are a friendly, "green" way to clear the air. Just seeing the plants may stimulate a sense of well-being. One study of surgery patients showed quicker recovery rates when their hospital rooms gave a view of a garden or an area with trees.

It is suggested that maximum air purification comes when you have a minimum of one plant for every 100 square feet of living space. Don't worry about overestimating—the more the better, especially if you have central heat and air. The plants will help control the humidity of your living space, absorbing the humidity when it's thick in the air, releasing it when it's dry. That adds up to you being more comfortable—and energized.

To get the best humidity control from your plants, keep them well watered but not drowned. Water them the way you need to be watered—when needed. This will keep your plants thriving and healthier than a massive watering once a week. They also need more water in the winter when the humidity is low, just as you do. A good watering can do you both a world of good.

Water: The Energy Enhancer

Too tired for that walk? It may be hard to believe, but the number-one factor in fatigue is dehydration. If you do nothing else in your quest for weight loss but begin to drink water each day—and drink a lot of it—you will experience a phenomenal boost in your energy and sense of well-being. Few of my clients think of water as their most important energy enhancer, yet many of the symptoms of fatigue that we blame on too much stress and too little sleep are simply the result of thirst.

At the end of a long workday, when you feel rotten and headachy and unwilling to exercise—in a strange zone between sore and numb—your body is crying out to be hydrated. Chances are you've only drunk enough water to wash down a few aspirin and have had little else since that coffee or diet soda this morning. You've been breathing dry, air-conditioned or heated air at the office, and the chronic stress in your routine has caused some moments of intense perspiration. And of course, you've been losing fluids during the day through normal body functions—fluids that haven't been replaced. You're parched!

Water is important for your energy metabolism for several vital reasons. Consider that your body is composed primarily of water: It's 92 percent of your blood plasma, 80 percent of your muscle mass, 60 percent of your red blood cells, and 50 percent of everything else in your body. Every cell in your body relies on water to dilute biochemicals, vitamins, and minerals to just the right concentrations. Your body also depends on the bloodstream to transport nutrients and other substances from one part to another, and this too depends on optimal fluid concentration. Blood volume actually decreases and "thickens" when you are dehydrated, meaning that the heart has to work harder to supply your body with needed oxygen. And remember, oxygenated blood is the key for effective energy metabolism.

Water is also vital for maintaining proper muscle tone, allowing muscles to contract naturally and increase in mass. When dehydrated, the muscles are more injury-prone and will not work to optimal performance. In fact, dehydrated muscles will only work to 30 or 35 percent of their capacity. This spells mediocre performance for athletes, tiredness, achiness, and headaches for you, and an inability to build body muscle while losing body fat. Without oxygen getting to the cells, fat cannot be burned for energy.

Drink Yourself Well

Drinking more water is a challenge for most of us. Most Americans have grown up drinking just about anything but water. We list our favorite beverages as soda, coffee, tea, juice, but delegate water only to washing down pills, washing away dirt, and brushing teeth.

Water is an essential nutrient. Without food, a person can survive (although not well) for days, even months. But without water, the human body can survive only three to five days.

Again, water is a metabolic booster because it is a critical component of basic functions for your body's health. First, along with proper protein and salt intake, water works to release excess stores of fluid, much like priming a pump. It is the natural diuretic. No other beverage works like water to prevent the body from holding excess fluids. Second, water transports the energy nutrients throughout your body and is essential for maintaining your body temperature. Third, water helps you digest food and maintains proper bowel function and waste elimination. Being a mild laxative, water actually activates the fiber you eat, allowing it to form a bulky mass that passes through the gastrointestinal tract easily and quickly. Without proper water, fiber becomes a difficult-to-pass "glue" in your colon. Big water-drinkers get less colon and bladder cancer.

Water is the only liquid we consume that doesn't require the body to work to metabolize or excrete it. Even fresh juices do not provide the solid benefits of pure, wonderful water, since your body must process the substances they contain. With soft drinks, your body has to work overtime to process and excrete the chemicals and colorings. Although based on water, sodas are "polluted" water.

Many other beverages, particularly those with caffeine, actually remove more water than contained in the beverage itself. Coffee, tea, and some sodas contain tannic acid, a product that interferes with iron and calcium absorption and competes for excretion with other bodily waste products such as uric acid. When not properly excreted, this uric acid can build up in the body and crystallize around the joints. This build-up leads to joint pain in elbows, shoulders, knees, and feet, especially former injury spots, and is a type of gouty arthritis. Men are particularly prone to uric acid excesses. This is one reason why a cup of tea or coffee, although fluid based, just doesn't do the job. Furthermore, water works to lubricate joints.

If you're still not convinced about the wonders of water, consider this: Water also works to keep the skin healthy, resilient, and wrinkle-resistant. It could honestly be labeled an "anti-aging" ingredient!

How Much Do I Need?

The answer: Eight to ten eight-ounce glasses each day—more when you exercise, travel by plane, or live at high altitudes. Sound overwhelming? Never thirsty? You're not alone. This water prescription brings out cries of anguish from many people.

But you really do need that much because you lose that much every day. Your body continually loses water as it performs necessary functions. Even breathing uses up your fluid stores; every time you exhale, you blow off water—to the tune of about two cups per day. Water evaporates from your skin to cool your body, even when you aren't aware of sweating. These losses, along with what is lost in regular urination and bowel movements, total up to ten cups per day. When perspiring heavily, the amount lost can double or triple.

Take heart! As you begin to meet your body's needs by drinking more water, your natural thirst will increase. You may find water drinking habit-forming; the more you drink, the more you want.

Start increasing your intake any way you can: through a straw, in a sports sipper, from a silver pitcher. Add fresh lemon or lime, drink sparkling water, buy bottled water—just drink it! Try filling a two-quart container with water each morning, and then make sure it's all gone before you go to bed. I also encourage drinking a twelve- to sixteen-ounce glass of water right after each meal and snack throughout the day. If you are eating as often as you should, every three hours or so, this will provide a large proportion of the fluid you need.

Tips for Staying Hydrated

Start Your Day With Eight to Sixteen Ounces of Water

While the coffee or tea is brewing, drink a cup or two of water. You wake up with a water deficit, so drinking water soon after waking will gently restore hydration. Many of my clients swear by a cup of warm water with a squeeze of lemon first thing in the morning to jump-start their digestive system gently. They declare it's the answer to their "regularity" problems.

Get Your Eight a Day

This isn't a diet principle; it's just how your body is wired. Take water breaks routinely, at least every thirty-five to forty-five minutes, even more frequently when the air is dry or hot. Try to drink little or nothing with your meals (sip water if you must), because washing food down with water dilutes the digestive function.

Get More When You Need It

You may not automatically know when you need more, but look for the subtle signs of dehydration—dry eyes, nose or mouth, impatience, slight nausea, flushed skin, dizziness, headaches, weakness, and mild fatigue. Also, drink when you're more stressed than normal. Not to make you obsessive, but it's a good idea to glance at your urine occasionally. Other than first thing in the morning, a dark yellow color is a sign your kidneys are having to concentrate the waste in too-small a volume of liquid. Pale-colored urine indicates good hydration.

Don't Wait Until You're Thirsty to Drink

It's already too late. Once you feel thirsty, you've already lost a significant amount of fluid. So don't rely on your thirst mechanism. It will prompt you to replace only 35 to 40 percent of your body's hydration needs. And if you don't take in adequate water, your body fluids will be thrown out of balance and you may experience fluid retention, constipation, unexplained weight gain, and a greater malfunction in your natural thirst mechanism.

Keep Water Where You Are

You're more apt to keep up with water needs if you keep drinking water close at hand. Freeze large bottles of water overnight and pull them out in the morning. The water thaws through the day, but is still chilled. Keep a glass or a pitcher of water at your desk, and refill it often. At home, keep a pitcher or large bottle of water in the refrigerator, with a glass on the counter as a reminder.

Avoid Dehydrating Food and Drinks

Caffeine-containing and alcoholic beverages act as dehydrators, further increasing, and never replacing, your fluid needs. In fact, each cup of coffee or tea adds an extra cup of water to the eight-to-ten-a-day basic requirement. Who has the room—or time?

Fill Up Before You Work Out—And Keep It Up!

Drink sixteen ounces of water fifteen to thirty minutes before your workout. Avoid starting to exercise when you're already thirsty; you're guaranteed a substandard performance. Continue to fill up while you're working out. Drink six to eight ounces of water every twenty minutes during your workout or training. This may seem like a lot, but even this doesn't begin to keep up with typical sweat losses. When possible, drink cool water—it is absorbed into the system more quickly. No need for a sports drink to replenish electrolytes unless you're exercising longer than ninety minutes.

Practice Air Travel Smarts

Drink as if you're going into an exercise workout: sixteen ounces before your flight, then at least eight more every hour aloft. Stick with water or juices.

If You Start Craving Salt, Go for Water

Once your fluid stores drop below a certain level, your thirst mechanism cuts off altogether. (Possibly to preserve your sanity if you're lost in the desert?) What turns on is a desire for salt—or salty foods. It's one of those magnificent things the body does: because extra sodium holds more fluids in the body, the salt craving is a survival mechanism to slow life-threatening dehydration. Notice a craving for hot dogs and nachos at the beach? Look for a water bottle instead.

Is Tap Water Okay?

Be sure not to let the bottled versus tap versus treated water controversy get in the way of your health. Many people do; they don't trust their tap water, so they drink no water at all.

Public water systems today are well monitored for safety, and bottled water companies are now beginning to fall under similar standards. You can assure yourself of the purity and safety of your local drinking water by checking with your local EPA or health department, or by contacting EPA's Safe Drinking Water Hotline at 800-426-4791. If you lack confidence in the answers you receive, you can have your water tested privately. The agencies listed above can give you the names of testing laboratories.

If you drink bottled water, choose brands that bottle their water in glass or clear plastic containers and are able and willing to provide an analysis or certification of purity. And buy only spring or purified water—a bottle labeled "drinking water" may just come from your municipal water system. You would do just as well turning on your faucet.

The biggest concern with tap water is that it is treated with chlorine to remove contaminants. As important as chlorine is for purifying our water, questions have been raised about its contribution to heart disease risk, to miscarriage, and to long-term effects on the immune system. I encourage my clients to avoid, when possible, water that has an obvious taste or smell of chlorine. When you travel, consider ordering bottled water.

You may want to get information on a water-purifying system for your home. Steam distillation is the most reliable, and most expensive, form of filtration. The next best is reverse osmosis, which forces the water through a cellophane-like, semipermeable membrane that acts as a barrier to contaminants like asbestos, copper, lead, mercury, and even some microorganisms. Reverse osmosis systems require a good bit of water pressure to function and are often difficult to access for necessary filter changes. And the replacement filters can be quite expensive.

Activated carbon filters use granules, precoat (a fine powder), or a solid block to remove unpleasant odors, colors, and bad tastes from drinking water, and do a very good job in removing chlorine and some contaminants. If all you're after is good taste and less chlorine odor and aren't concerned about microorganisms or other contaminants, a simple table-top pitcher with a carbon filter (such as Brita) will suffice. If you drink tap water, the taste may improve after refrigerating it for twenty-four hours (the chlorine will dissipate). This can be a low-cost way to get the more refreshing taste of bottled water without the cost. Your choice of which water to drink comes down to taste, cost, and availability.

Regardless, the bottom line is this: Drink eight to ten glasses of water every day, and more if you exercise heavily. Don't allow anything to become a substitute for the beverage your body likes best: water, the beverage of champions!

CHAPTER 6

S
M
A
REST
T

FOR SOME OF US, IT'S AS DIFFICULT to turn off the day as it is to turn off the TV. There is simply too much to do and not enough time to do it, and robbing from sleep seems an easy way to make up the difference. Ask ten people how disciplined they are with a sleep schedule and you'll likely hear variations on a single theme: "I go to bed when I finish doing what I have to do." Bombarded by increasing demands on their time from work, travel, play, family, and social obligations, most people steal time from sleep. In fact, some are downright proud of undersleeping. Getting by on four hours has a superhuman sound.

A National Sleep Foundation survey found nearly two out of three people do not get the recommended eight hours of sleep each night. A third of those get less than six hours of sleep. Other surveys have shown that in the past year, one-third of American adults have had trouble falling asleep or staying asleep and two-thirds complained of sleep-related problems such as insomnia, snoring, or restless legs. The late hours designated for rest mirror our days: we fight through them.

Sleep and Your Health

Sleep is a little known and often missed component in the weight-loss game: a bad night's sleep might do more than give you the early-morning blues; it can actually play a central role in locking down your fat cells. Results from studies of the impact of sleep deprivation on the body indicate that a chronic lack of sleep may affect metabolic function as much as living a sedentary lifestyle. Being consistently deprived of sleep can also increase the severity of age-related chronic disorders, including diabetes, obesity, and hypertension.

Sleep is the repair shop of the body and brain, the process that most thoroughly restores our psychological and physiological vitality after the strain and exertion of life. Along with building and repairing our muscle tissue, bones, cells, and immune system, restful sleep allows the release of important hormones such as the human growth hormone, which is critical for vitality and metabolic burn.

Sleep researchers have shown that cheating on sleep for only one night increases evening cortisol to levels that can adversely impact health by lowering immune responses and slowing the body's fat-burning potential. Because cortisol helps to regulate blood sugar concentrations, the sleep-deprived body metabolizes glucose less effectively. Increased levels of cortisol can also damage brain cells, causing shrinkage in the hippocampus, the critical region of the brain that regulates learning.

Small sleep losses can be cumulative. Research has revealed that after even one week's lack of sleep, there are striking alterations in metabolic and endocrine function and a rapid deterioration of the body's functions. The good news is that these studies also show that the negative effects of sleep deprivation can be corrected by normal sleep. Just as a lack of sleep can harm the body, getting sleep can help it.

How Much Is Enough?

Research still shows that the average adult needs seven-and-a-half to eight hours of deep, restful sleep a night to stay healthy and alert. There are exceptions: one in ten needs ten hours of sleep each night, one in one hundred can be refreshed with five. Again, new studies show that cutting back on sleep to below the seven-and-a-half hours most of us need can be as dangerous to health as a poor diet and no exercise.

There appears to be a biological feedback loop between the body's use of energy, its need to resupply it, and the brain's mechanism for maintaining the proper energy balance. This need of the brain for energy helps to explain why lack of sleep dulls the brain, saps energy, increases irritability and depression, and turns up the appetite thermostat. We think we can lose sleep and be a little tired, but otherwise we'll be just fine. The truth is we won't—we ultimately have to pay the piper. We may be living life in the modern age, but we still have the same bodies, living by the same principles, that we were created with.

ABC's of Good ZZZ's

If it's a little harder for you to shut off the business of your mind than it is to shut off the light, you may need some tips for sweet sleep. Rather than endure one more sleepless night or another morning dragging out of bed, use these tips to program your body for restful sleep. The bottom line: How well you live your day impacts how well you sleep at night.

Be Clock-Driven

When it comes to catching up on lost sleep, timing is everything. Block in sleep as a priority part of your schedule. By doing this you are making the decision that sleep is important because being your very best is important.

Your body's internal time clock is daily reset by getting up at the same time each day. "Sleeping in," even for an hour, can disrupt your biological clock and end up making you feel even more fatigued. This is why getting to bed earlier in the evening is better than sleeping late

SLEEP ROBBERS

If you desire more sleep, but your body simply won't cooperate, check this list of likely suspects that may be stealing your much-needed rest.

Blood Sugar Fluctuations. Sleep deprivation and the resulting cortisol production cause your blood sugar level to fluctuate. In turn, blood sugar fluctuations are a prime culprit in restless sleep. A sudden drop in your blood sugar level, characteristically occurring at 2:30 to 3 A.M., causes a surge in adrenaline. This can bring on a panic response, which is why you often wake with a start, with your heart and mind racing. Once awakened, it's difficult to get back to restful sleep.

Hot Flashes and Night Sweats. The results of blood sugar crashes, menopause, and panic attacks last only a few minutes but are notorious for disrupting sleep. If they are hormone related and you're a female approaching menopause, please don't ignore the hormone issue. Let troublesome hot flashes and night sweats motivate you to consider hormone replacement therapy or healing soy foods.

Getting Older. It's a myth that you need less sleep as you age. But your sleep patterns will likely change. You may sleep less in one stretch. You also get less of the deeper, most restorative sleep. Consequently, you awaken more often and are more easily aroused by a snoring spouse or a call to the bathroom.

the next morning—it gives you the extra rest without upsetting your rhythm. Stick with it. People who are just starting to make up lost sleep can take six weeks to recover fully.

I know this is hard, but try to get up at the same time every day, regardless of when you fall asleep. Set your alarm clock—then put it out of sight. You want to be clock-driven, not clock-obsessed.

Choose Nighttime Snacks Wisely

Overeating, or eating high-fat, high-sugar snacks after dinner can so overload your body that it will resist getting to sleep or staying asleep. The classic pattern is being awakened around 3:00 A.M., eyes open, heart racing, unable to get back to sleep. Eating too much too

Stress. It's the top cause of short-term sleep problems due to the chemical gymnastics it causes in your body. Just worrying about your insomnia can worsen the problem.

Medications. Steroids and some drugs can disrupt sleep. The most common troublemakers are some blood pressure medications, diet pills, diuretics, antidepressants, cold and allergy remedies, and asthma medications. Check with your physician and pharmacist.

Caffeine. Americans drink 400 million cups of coffee each day, and get extra doses of caffeine in tea or cola-type sodas, cocoa, and chocolate. Caffeine's stimulants are still at work five to seven hours after you've ingested it, preventing your body from falling into deep sleep and often awakening you prematurely by disrupting sleep patterns.

A Nightcap or Night Smoke. Alcohol in the bloodstream makes staying asleep more difficult. In addition, it suppresses dreams, depriving your body of its normal, refreshing sleep cycle. Nicotine is a stimulant that keeps your body from easily falling asleep. One more reason to kick the habit!

Illness. Arthritis, asthma, and sleep apnea (breathing cessation characterized by loud snoring and gasping) can interfere with sleep. Depression can also cause insomnia, just as insomnia can bring on depression.

late has put your body into chemical gymnastics. Going to bed hungry can be a sleep-robbing culprit as well. When you're hungry your brain will try to keep you alert until you eat.

A great bedtime snack is a small bowl of whole-grain cereal with low-fat milk or half a turkey sandwich or a banana with skim milk. All help keep the body chemistries properly balanced through the night, allowing you to waken rested and refreshed.

Work Your Body During the Day

Exercise, with its ability to process the stressors of our day physically, gives sweeter sleep; it's nature's best tranquilizer! People who work out for thirty to forty minutes, four times a week, fall asleep faster and sleep longer than nonexercisers. Just don't exercise less than an hour before bedtime—the rise in your body temperature can keep you awake.

Keep It Cool, Dark, and Quiet

People sleep best in rooms that are between 60 and 65 degrees, pitch-black, and silent. If that's a far cry from your bedroom, put up heavy draperies or a light-blocking shade. To drown out traffic noises or a snoring spouse, try wearing ear plugs or adding "white noise" like a fan or air-conditioner.

Check Your Nighttime Posture

One of the often overlooked causes of daytime fatigue is nighttime posture. Sleeping on your stomach can cause a strain on your back that might be just painful enough to keep you from getting a good night's sleep. For the most restful repose night after night, sleep on your side. This promotes easier breathing and reduces snoring, which can wake you up. Consider keeping a pillow under your knees; this comfortably flexes your lower spine, making it say "ahhhh...." To avoid neck and shoulder aches, use a pillow that's low enough to support your head without flexing your neck. Down pillows work best; foam ones are often too springy. And be sure you're warm enough: If you have to stay curled up all night to keep warm, your back is likely to get sore.

Develop a Sleep Ritual

Remember the bedtime story that helped to calm you down as a child? An adult bedtime routine gives your brain strong cues that it's time to slow down and prepare for sleep. It can be as simple or as elaborate as you like—a warm bath, lighting a candle (particularly a calming lavender one), putting a "brow pillow" on your forehead, snuggling up with your loved one, or listening to classical music. (Just ten minutes of Mozart has been shown to rein in the racing mind—for both sleep and performance.)

Some people are avid writers before bed, particularly when their mind is racing. Writing down what you're thinking and feeling helps to "drain the brain" for restful sleep. I have more than a few clients who lie down for five minutes, then get up and make a to-do list, writing down everything that needs to be attended to the next day. Then they set it aside, and set aside time the next day to deal with their list.

Let Bed Be Bed

Don't let it be an office, a place to pay bills, or a home theater. Make your bed restful by using it only for sleeping and romance.

Don't force the sleep issue. If you're still awake thirty minutes after going to bed, get up and do something calming, such as reading, until you're groggy enough to fall asleep. Try to stay awake until your eyes close involuntarily. This works best if you don't keep track of time.

Other Bright Ideas, Like ...Light!

Sunlight is the "spark of life," without which there would be no plant growth, no photosynthesis, no oxygen. On a more personal level, light causes normal physiological fluctuations that can affect the way we feel, think, and sleep. Depending on personal sensitivity and the extent of light changes in your environment, the effects can range from mild fatigue to severe depression.

What keeps us tied to light is a cleverly balanced internal clock, known as circadian rhythm, which synchronizes a variety of physiological systems including heart rate, body temperature, and sleep cycles. This internal clock is set by light; it can be reset by changes in the timing or duration of light exposure.

Most of us don't think twice about our circadian rhythms. We take for granted that we become tired and sleepy at night, awake and alert during the day. We notice the effects only if our internal clock is "out of sync." Most people notice the effects of circadian rhythms when they gain or lose time while traveling or during seasonal changes in light. Even small changes can cause dramatic symptoms in some people.

To help smooth out your sleep/wake cycle, try these simple measures to manipulate your exposure to light:

- If you get up in the middle of the night, avoid turning on bright lights. Light suppresses melatonin production and may make it more difficult to fall back to sleep. Put dimmer switches or nightlights in bathrooms and hallways.
- If you have trouble rising in the morning, maximize the amount of light in your bedroom as soon as you wake up.
- If you wake up too early in the morning, minimize the amount of dawn light. Wear a sleep mask or put blackout shades on your windows. When you wake, keep lights dim to help gradually shift your usual pattern.

In all of creation, the principle of rest is modeled for us. The soil of the earth needs a rest from time to time, allowing it to become more productive. Bears hibernate, fish sleep with their eyes open, the most beautiful plants have a period of dormancy. Our needs are no different: We need rest in order to heal and rejuvenate. So treat yourself well. Give yourself time to recharge and replenish so you can keep your metabolism burning brightly.

CHAPTER 7

S

M

A

R

TREATING YOURSELF WELL

THE LIVES OF SO MANY OF US are two-dimensional—work and food. Doing and eating. It's hard to find a place for relaxation and replenishment—sometimes even personal relationships. You know you should spend more quality time on yourself but just thinking about how to fit it in gives you a migraine. It's easier just to hit the sofa—take in some food and tune out with TV.

Many of us push ourselves into prolonged periods of exertion without adequate periods of rest and relaxation. Some of us push ourselves through long days with barely time for a bathroom break, and definitely no time for lunch. Some go months, even years, without a vacation, or a relaxing weekend. No wonder we get run down, and robbed of the joy and peace we so desire.

This breakneck pace not only inflates your stress level, but takes a hefty toll on your metabolism and your quality of life. It signals the body to eat, and overeat, in order to provide the energy to keep up with the demands of your daily grind, yet slows you down to conserve what energy you do have. When life borders on depletion, food (and storing that food) takes center stage. Losing weight becomes impossible.

If you are approaching meltdown, the best thing to do, ironically, is nothing at all. You were created with a need to rest, to recreate, to reflect, and to be regenerated. Treating yourself well is really a lifestyle. It makes a statement that "you deserve a break today."

Here are some ways to achieve a wiser, saner, and metabolically boosted you.

Chill Out!

Countless studies have documented the benefits of chilling out. Anything that relieves stress also boosts physical, spiritual, and emotional energy and becomes a metabolic booster. Fatigue disappears; backaches vanish; colds and flu are kept at bay; blood pressure drops; and chronic conditions—such as migraine, irritable bowel syndrome, insomnia, even acne—improve.

Sure, it used to be a little easier to get a break. Fifteen years ago, most stores were not open on Sundays. Now, Sunday is a day for shopping. The notion of the Sabbath being a day of rest has disappeared. You can go to the all-night supermarket and get your entire week's food at 3 A.M. And holidays—even those like Labor Day and New Year—are a merchant's delight, a time for some of the biggest clearance sales of the year.

To really enjoy life physically, emotionally, relationally, and spiritually, we must have a way, and take the time, to recharge our physical batteries and renew our spirits. Here's how.

Make a Date With Yourself

At least once a week, carve out one hour (or longer) for your own— an hour in which you have nothing to do. Plan ahead on when the hour will be, but don't plan what you'll do—otherwise it will

TRIM YOUR CALENDAR

Just because you *can* do everything doesn't mean that you *must* do everything. Ruthlessly cross out unnecessary events in your calendar. Time pressure is a huge metabolism zapper. Research tells us that although we feel more rushed and harried than we did twenty or thirty years ago, we actually have more free time than we used to. We just feel pressured to do more because of our super-speedy culture. E-mail, laptops, and cell phones create the illusion that we can, and should, be busy and productive every minute of the day.

While you can't always stop responsibilities from piling up, you can pick what requires immediate attention and what can be put on the back burner. So go ahead, cancel some social events and some not-so-vital work commitments and do exactly what you want. It will energize you beyond words and remove a major logjam to your metabolic burn.

become one more thing on your "to-do" list.

I actually try to spend one day a week in timeout rest, whether it's Sunday or another day. I need a consistent weekly withdrawal to do replenishing activities. A day of rest for me means a day of activities that personally revitalize me. It may mean reading novels, taking leisurely walks, napping, enjoying friends, window shopping, or just sitting, daydreaming, and writing.

For some people, this kind of activity would provoke anxiety. To relax and be replenished, they need to be skydiving, or driving a race car! And that's fine—"relaxing" means different things to different people. But just switching to a different activity, even if it's physically strenuous, can revive you. Studies have shown that curiosity increases our performance capability. When devoid of stimulation, people become disorganized, lose their intellectual ability to concentrate, and decline in coordination. So read a new book, paint your masterpiece, and seek out new situations, work opportunities, and challenges. We are stimulus-hungry beings, and denying our nature can lead to inertia and listlessness.

Does all this sound more like the ideal than reality? It needn't be. This is a great time to carve out our personal hours of renewal, because living in contemporary society has made our need desperate. With determination and a little creativity, anyone can make the time for timeout.

Something happens to me when I choose to relax and be replenished. I return to what I was created to be: a human being. With time invested in recharging, I can review how I'm normally spending my time and reevaluate according to the purposes that have been placed in my heart. Otherwise, I stay too busy for issues of the soul.

Start Your Day With a Timeout

Many of us have learned the power of starting the morning with a quiet time of reflection and spiritual connection. This is a daily part of my life because I know that I could be doing nothing more important, and that it is the only way to start my day with strength. It is a timeout in the midst of my busyness to reflect on what my source of strength really is, who I really am, and that nothing, NOTHING, is worth being robbed of the joy of life. Starting my day with quiet reflection is like the warm-up for my exercise—a time to stretch spiritually and get my soul circulating.

I get up and eat breakfast (body fuel) while reading inspirational words (soul fuel). Then, I walk. While walking, I'm also reflecting— not just going through a mental checklist and to-do list, but taking a step beyond to look at the "why" of my life: What's the passion, what's the purpose, why am I doing all these things, and why am I spinning all these plates? Sometimes I need to focus more on what I need to say no to, more than on what to say yes to. After this time of listening and reflecting, writing is my way to get my thoughts and feelings into a place where I can take action. Writing down what's inside is a ten-minute investment that yields huge dividends for me.

More Breaks, More Breakthroughs

Research shows that no matter how busy people are, they would work better, faster, and more productively if they took a break. True, withdrawing from your endeavors for a few moments temporarily halts your output, but research shows that doing so can erase tension, enhance optimistic attitudes, focus the mind, jump-start creativity, and give a significant energy and metabolic boost. Why work hours on end at a slightly unfocused 75 percent performance, when a fifteen-minute power break can help you work at an efficient 100 percent for the next few hours?

And that's exactly what happens. Research shows that after every few hours of focused activity, your brain and body take a downturn. Blood sugars begin to drop, energy levels fade, alertness dims, and metabolism slows. You need to get up, get a snack, get water, get moving, and get your mind off the work. If you ignore this need, or try to shake it off, you'll only achieve a lower level of productivity.

You may need to write breaks into your schedule as a priority appointment—as important as any other. It is that important. Even the busiest people—a surgeon doing open-heart surgeries, a judge hearing back-to-back cases—can manipulate their difficult schedules to allow for break time. If you realize how important it is, you can make it happen. Remember this: More breaks, more breakthroughs!

Using your break for a power nap can also be very refreshing— relaxing your body, clearing your mind, improving your mood, and boosting your energy levels. Studies show that you don't really have to sleep to get the rejuvenation you need—just shut the door, unplug the phone, turn off the lights, and close your eyes. Rest and be replenished. Then get up and have a power snack. Stretch or take a quick walk at the end of your break to rejuvenate yourself for the work at hand.

If you choose to nap, make it short and sweet. Don't tell toddlers this, but a fifteen- to twenty-minute nap seems to be ideal for the maximum energy boost. You can stretch it a few extra minutes, but don't go over an hour. Napping too long can be counterproductive; long naps can allow you to enter into the deeper delta-type sleep, causing a groggy, disoriented state when you wake that takes a long time to snap out of. If you seem to need more than an hour's nap in the afternoon, you're probably not getting enough sleep at night.

End Your Day With a Timeout

I have recently begun to end my day with a timeout. This is very difficult for me; I have to tell myself more than once that there is nothing more I should be doing. I then enjoy some of my favorite things that don't seem very productive in the scheme of life, yet I know are vital to recharge my energy: reading travel magazines, listening to favorite music, whatever.

Again, it doesn't come naturally for me; I'm a "doer" by nature. The first one up in our household, I go nonstop till the sun goes down and beyond. Even my "breaks" have often been purposeful: planning, researching, meeting with a small group. I have laughed for many years about being a "human doing" rather than a "human being," but only in recent years have I realized it's not something to laugh about. Ending my day with a time just to "be" reaffirms in my own mind that I am only human—and that's more than enough!

Extend Timeouts Twice a Year

I try to begin each year with a personal retreat, a time to write and reflect on where I've been and where I'm going. Is it the direction I want, propelling me toward my dreams?

I try to take another time to pull away midyear to do a midpoint check. What have the past six months done to me and for me? Am I on track with the goals and priorities I established six months earlier? Am I treating myself well—and honoring my body, soul, and beliefs?

At least twice a year, schedule time to pull away and completely change your scenery. Even if it's only for a weekend, physically separating yourself from your daily obligations can do a world of good for your energy level. Leaving your familiar environment is a surefire way to recharge and refresh your batteries. Viewing life in a new context is itself invigorating. When you return, you'll have a new perspective.

Let your time away build your motivation for making your day-to-day world more beautiful, more relaxing—and definitely more energizing. Treating yourself well is more than just taking action—it is a state of mind, a state of soul. You can enter into rest anytime you choose to let go of all the stuff you don't want, won't use, and don't need. You feel uplifted and drawn to the new because you aren't struggling to carry the old.

Make Change

Embracing The Smart Weigh will work wonders with your metabolism and well-being—and it will bring something else into life: change. We humans are prone to fall into ruts in life—in the way we eat, the way we live, the way we interact with others. These ruts may provide safety, but they also bring boredom and weariness. So shake things up! Taking different actions will give you a different point of view, and that will remind you that you're in control of your choices and can change things for the better.

You probably have a suitcase full of habits and ruts that you aren't even aware of. By becoming conscious of them and then breaking or altering them, you can stir up your old thought patterns and emerge from your slump. Consider moving the furniture; mix up your schedule of doing things in the morning; do your work in a different location; eat a different breakfast; listen to some new music; cross-train in exercise; take a new route to the office or school; change the lighting; paint a room; try some unfamiliar fruits and vegetables.

The power of rearranging one's external environment has been well documented in studies since the 1960s. For years, Weight Watchers and other eating modification groups have used this strategy to help countless people lose weight by modifying their behavior and "stimulus environment." For example, external changes like eating from smaller plates or eating only at the table with a place mat—even just rearranging the refrigerator—can have a huge impact on the inside of you.

You will see how all these truths operate as you learn to make them a part of your daily life through the seven-week plan in the next chapter. Let it become the beginning of a new way of living!

CHAPTER 8

MAKING THE SMART WEIGH *YOUR* WAY: SEVEN WEEKS TO SUCCESS

NOW IT'S TIME TO PUT THE principles of The Smart Weigh into action—life-changing action. The first step is to set a realistic weight loss goal within an appropriate amount of time—about one pound per week. Accept that healthful weight loss is slow and steady. If you want to lose weight and keep it off, you have to change your behavior and eating habits permanently. But you don't have to do it all at once. Make small changes, like walking two or three days a week, cutting out frequent desserts—things you can achieve without much trouble. The key is setting goals you can achieve. That reinforces a positive feeling that helps you go on. And success breeds success.

Building a Healthy Foundation

The Smart Weigh offers week-by-week suggestions to help you change your lifestyle in a way that releases your body's natural ability to lose weight. Each week's suggestions build on what you have done in the previous week; after seven weeks, you will have created the foundation of a healthy lifestyle—one that places you on The Smart Weigh. This exclusive plan combines the best of the best: it combines every top strategy shown by research to increase your chances of reaping the joys of fitness and good health.

There is no need to do this plan in just seven weeks. You may

PLAN FOR *SUCCESS*

SET YOUR GOALS

Decide what changes you want to make, keeping in mind that you should be specific and realistic. "Lose weight" is a broadly defined goal. A more specific and realistic goal would be, "Lose ten pounds within two months." The key word here is *realistic*—try achieving a comfortable weight you maintained easily as a young adult. Write down your goals and then let others know about them. That will increase the likelihood that you'll follow through and get support when you need it.

UNDERSTAND YOUR PASSIONS

Lose weight because you want to, not to please someone else. You must want to lose weight because it's what you want to do. Know what really makes you feel good, what you like to do, and use that to help guide you to your long-term goals. This step requires you to narrow your focus to one or two specific goals. Which goals do you value most? These will become your priorities.

CRITICALLY PLAN YOUR STEPS

Determine small steps that will lead to the larger one. If you want to drop ten pounds, follow the guides for weight loss that will bring your calories down and your nutrition up. Exercise appropriately to come up with a 500-calorie-a-day deficit. This will allow you to lose the weight in one-pound or two-pound increments per week.

CHALLENGE YOURSELF

Realize that if you want to lose weight, you might feel discontented sometimes, or feel a little out of breath while working out. Acknowledge that change is not easy. If it were, you would have already accomplished your goal. When want to slow the pace and incorporate the principles over the next seven months, or even over the next year. Remember, it has taken you a lifetime to accumulate your current habits and attitudes; it will take longer than a few weeks to weed out the negative ones, plant new ones, and allow them to grow into a new you. Of course, I have many clients who are the all-or-nothing type people, and they make

things get difficult, we tend to revert to previous comfortable behaviors. But now is the time to develop new lifestyle behaviors. To do that, you have to change the behaviors that resulted in weight gain in the first place. Lifestyle changes involve taking a realistic, sometimes painfully honest look at your eating habits and daily routine. Were you taught as a child to clean your plate? If so, do you still feel compelled to eat everything, even when you're full? Examine your eating style. Do you eat fast? Do you take big bites? When do you eat? While watching television? All the time? Examine your shopping and cooking techniques.

Evaluate Your Progress

Are you making headway? If not, why not? Adjust your plan to meet your long-term goal. Are you meeting your weekly or monthly weight-loss goals? If not, determine what the problem might be. Do you need more consistency with exercise? Do you need to be eating more often—or become more careful with portion sizes?

Stay Focused

That means not being deterred by obstacles that threaten to obscure your goal. Are you invited to a great party where there's lots of food? Look past the buffet table and envision yourself as the fit and trim person you want to be. That should help you control yourself.

Savor Your Accomplishments

Reward yourself for reaching small goals along the way. As you lose weight and become more fit, buy yourself some new clothes. Have you developed a pleasant routine of walking? Treat yourself to a walk on the beach or around a lake.

a total about-face and dive into the whole seven-week plan the very first day. But, as I've said before, these truths are simple, but they are not easy. Give yourself time to succeed, and resist the notion that you've failed—what I call the "I've Already Blown It" Syndrome—if you veer off course for a meal or a day.

Even when you succumb to temptation and consume foods you know interfere with your health, be assured that a lapse in healthy eating doesn't ruin all the health you have attained over weeks of wellness. A lapse is just that—a lapse. Don't let it become a relapse, another relapse, and finally a collapse. Look at each meal and snack as an event—don't wrap it all into one bad day or one unhealthy weekend. Instead, get right back on track with the next meal or snack. Your body will stabilize quickly, you'll feel great, and you'll be thanking yourself the next day.

Read over the seven-week plan, then set a date to begin, a date to embrace a new way of living—for life. Over the course of the seven-week plan, you'll do what few people do—you'll follow through on a vision and a commitment. Research tells us that it takes twenty-one days to break a habit, and thirty days to establish a new one. It takes forty days to start feeling comfortable with your new way of living. So your efforts during these seven weeks will work to start sealing your new behavior of eating, exercising, resting, and self-care into lifetime patterns. May your journey be one that leads you to a fulfilled life—body, soul, and spirit. May you be filled with good food, good health, and great joy!

Your Seven-Week Plan

Week One

Begin to eat early, often, and balanced; drink water, get moving, and get some sleep.

Action Steps
• Begin by following The Smart Weigh Jump-start Plan on page 28

- After the initial three days, begin a new food diary for the remainder of the week using the "Eat Right Prescription" to activate your metabolism (eat early, often, balanced, lean, and bright). This is a time to focus on what to eat rather than what to avoid. Have a balanced breakfast every day, and power snacks or meals every two and a half to three hours (see page 41 for power snack ideas or creatively put together your own). Also keep track of the eight to ten glasses of water you drink each day.

- Try to walk at least ten minutes a day for five days of this week. If you are already exercising aerobically at least four times a week, keep it up—and do the walk in addition.

- Look at your sleep patterns and the hours you invest in this vital key to wellness. If you aren't getting at least seven to eight hours of sleep each night, try to get to bed a bit earlier two nights this week.

Week Two

Be sure to eat early, often, and balanced—with special attention to eating lean and bright. Choose whole-grain foods, low-fat proteins, and a variety of brightly colored fruits and vegetables. Increase your exercise time, using it as a time to reflect and be refreshed. Breathe deeply and fully.

ACTION STEPS

- Compare your last week's food diary to the meal plan guidelines in the next chapter, and note adjustments you might want to make in timing or balance of eating. After you've evaluated your present-day eating habits and have found your weak spots, you can get on your way toward eating The Smart Weigh. Begin to eat in a focused way, using a goal-appropriate meal plan in Chapter 9 as your guide.

- This week, choose foods and portions for your meals and snacks based on your new plan. Keep in mind that these are guides for minimum portions and proper balance to achieve your desired goals for healthy living, putting you on the road to losing weight and feeling great. Get started with these amounts for the next two weeks to allow your body to stabilize before making adjustments, and keep a diary of what, when, and how much you eat and drink as well as exercise times and types, and how you feel. The diary on pages 218–221 provides space for you to list your protein choice, carbohydrates, and added fats.

- Increase walking to twenty minutes a day, either at one time or in two ten-minute sessions. If you are already exercising aerobically four times a week, do the twenty-minute walk on the other days.
- Begin to do the releasing/relaxing breathing described on page 97. Choose a time every day to practice your new focused breathing to release stress and breathe in life. Start with fifteen deep breaths at a time.

Week Three

Treat yourself well by eating well, exercising, resting, and making time for timeouts to reflect on your attitude and life purpose.

ACTION STEPS

- Review your day. Is there adequate time for timeouts? Carving out even ten minutes to reflect and be redirected is an excellent beginning. You may focus on writing this week as a way to study your thoughts. What negative thoughts about your progress seem to be recurring? What positive thoughts can you replace them with?
- Continue the breathing exercises. Practice the relaxing breath exercise whenever you feel anxious or upset, as well as at the beginning of your quiet time and exercise time. Try to have two focused breathing sessions each day.
- Treat yourself well by doing something nice for yourself: Go to a park or art museum, get a massage or pedicure. Or maybe just take a long, warm bath.
- Go through your pantry and refrigerator and aggressively remove the foods that no longer fit into your healthy lifestyle. Why keep them? Box up unopened cans and cake mixes and donate them to a local shelter for the disadvantaged. After planning your meals and snacks for the coming week, use The Smart Weigh grocery list on

pages 162–165 to shop smart. Pick up some fresh flowers to enjoy.
- Increase your walking to thirty minutes, at least five days this week. If you are doing another form of aerobic exercise, continue to walk on the other days.

Week Four

Use the dynamic duo of healthy eating and exercise to stabilize the rise and fall of your blood sugars and body chemistry.

ACTION STEPS
- Continue to choose foods and portions for your meals and snacks based on the meal plan that is appropriate for you. Review your food diary: Are there times of the day when you are hungry, or crave certain foods? How about your moods and energy? Are there times of the day when you are particularly high, or low? Adjust the timing of your eating to best stabilize your blood sugars. Also review your diaries for food choices that may contribute to better stabilization. For example, you may need to choose more of the best-choice whole grains and legumes on page 15.
- Check the mileage you are walking in your thirty minutes. If you are walking less than two miles, pick up your pace a bit. Continue exercising at least five days a week, and add in the conditioning exercises on pages 80–84 on two of the days.
- Choose four nights this week that you will go to bed early enough to get seven to eight hours of sleep. If you are waking up in the middle of the night, unable to get back to restful sleep, try a bowl of whole-grain cereal as your bedtime snack to stabilize your blood sugars through the night. Also review your day to be sure you are eating in even ways. Remember: How well you live your days affects how well you rest at night.

Week Five

Change your body physically by changing your environment and habits.

ACTION STEPS

- Do an activity outdoors, weather permitting. Even if it's a cloudy day you will still receive the serotonin-boosting effect of light. And warm up the indoor lights by changing the light bulbs, when possible, to a warm, incandescent light. Listen to some inspirational music during your quiet time or your walk, and do ten minutes of inspirational reading.

- Experiment with the meal ideas and recipes in Chapters 9 and 10 and break out of your rut! Add pizzazz by selecting at least three recipes you intend to try this week.

- Practice releasing/relaxing breathing for five minutes each day using the exercises on page 97 as your guide. Add in rhythmic two/one breathing.

- Continue to exercise, increasing your time to thirty-five minutes. Continue your conditioning work two days a week, and add in the flexibility exercises on pages 86–87 on two other days.

Week Six

Work toward proper portions of the foods you eat—and letting food be food: nourishment for your body. Slow down your eating and dine; don't inhale your meals.

ACTION STEPS

- How do you feel after eating? If you still feel hungry, or are craving something sweet, examine your food diary for the timing of the day's meal. Become a student of the setback; longer hours without eating will turn on your appetite and crank up cravings. Also, begin following The Ten Commandments of Satisfied Eating on pages 18–21.

- If you've not yet begun to journal, choose a day this week to write or reflect for ten minutes. Are your feelings fueling your appetite? What are some ways to express them that treat yourself well?

- Try some variety in your power snacks and breakfasts. Look at the "grab and go" suggestions in Chapter 10 for some fresh ideas.

- Continue to walk, increasing the time to forty minutes, five times a week. Check your heart rate and if you are not reaching your target zone for burning fat, pick up the pace and think about adding in some light (three-pound) hand-held weights, or cross-train, adding in some new activities. If you are doing another form of aerobic exercise, monitor your heart rate to stay in the fat-burning zone.

Week Seven

Eat power foods!. Try to include each food on the Nutritional Top Ten in your daily eating plan. Keep exercising, breathing, and taking care of yourself. Add a time to connect spiritually and to connect with others.

ACTION STEPS

- Review the Nutritional Top Ten on pages 56–57 and assess last week's eating. Are there immune-boosting power foods that you do not normally choose? Plan to include each of these foods in at least one meal or snack this week. You might begin with broccoli or salmon. If you are not a fish eater, plan to visit a natural foods store to pick up some flaxseed. Grind them, and sprinkle them over your cereal or salad. While shopping, look through the refrigerated and frozen sections to familiarize yourself with the many different products made from soybeans. Pick one to try as your protein source at a meal or as a snack.
- Add calisthenics to your aerobic, conditioning, and flexibility exercises. Use the abdominal exercises on pages 83–84 as a guide.
- Make a list of friends in whose company you feel more alive, happy, and optimistic. Pick one with whom to spend some time with this week.

The Big Picture

As you begin to make healthy changes in your lifestyle, be sure to keep your focus on the big picture of looking better and feeling better for life. You are not on a diet. You are choosing to take care of yourself and become the best you can be.

Ask yourself more important questions than just what weight you are striving for and how quickly you can get there. Ask yourself where you would like to be in the areas of:

Health: _____

Energy: _____

Mood: _____

Appearance: _____

Muscle Tone: _____

Weight: _____

Clothing Size: _____

Fitness Level: _____

Emotional Well-being: _____

Spirituality: _____

This is how one of my female clients answered these questions:

My Health: I want to stop getting sick every season—and lower my cholesterol and blood pressure.

My Energy: I want to wake up feeling energized and rested, and I want to have energy through my 3 P.M. slump time.

My Mood: I want to manage my moods, rather than allowing my moods to manage me. I no longer want to feel like "Ms. Jekyll/Ms. Hyde": positive one minute and cranky the next.

My Appearance: I want to have firmer skin, strong nails, shinier, fuller hair—and less fullness in my midsection.

My Muscle Tone: I want to get a "gravity" lift so that things aren't so saggy!

My Weight: I think I want and need to weigh about 148. I'm 5'7" and that's been a good weight for me in the past when I'm fit. But I really don't care about numbers on the scale as much as the size of my clothes.

My Clothing Size: I want to be back into size 8s and 10s again— I'm in big 12s and 14s now.

My Fitness Level: I want to be able to walk/run around the neighborhood and go up my stairs without getting winded.

My Emotional Well-Being: I want to feel emotions fully, and express them in healthy ways. I no longer want food to be my substitute for connecting with my own emotions or with others—I want to let food be food, not an emotional or relational gap-filler.

My Spirituality: I want to operate with a full spiritual tank—with a reservoir of peace and joy. I want to feel connected spiritually.

Climbing Beyond the Plateau

It sounds like bad news: Even the healthiest form of weight loss will result in weight plateaus. But it's actually good news—it's a sign your body is working right, and working for you. As you reach the body fat percentage where you have been in the past, your body attempts to adjust—as a survival mechanism—to keep you safe and secure at that historical weight. Metabolism will slow, blood sugars will fluctuate and you will hold fluids more readily, often masking the fat loss. If you hit a plateau, your goal is to stay the course of good eating and good exercise—putting strong focus onto the secrets for boosting your slowing metabolism up and over the plateau.

Ask yourself these questions:

1. Do you actually know what you are doing now? Have you gotten off track with timing, balance, or portions? Are you skipping meals to reduce caloric intake during the day and then overeating at night, thinking that it balances out?
2. Do you really need to lose more weight? Are you within the recommended weight range? Is it a body image problem affected by other things in your life that are "not right"? Or is it a body composition problem? A high percentage of body fat—say, 30 percent—even at an appropriate weight can mean the difference

of two clothing sizes larger than someone at the same given weight who has more muscle mass and just 20 percent body fat. Remember, your exercise is as vital as your eating in changing body composition.

3. Are you in a "rut?" Has your body become used to your current eating and exercise program? Is it time to "shake it up"?

Once you've answered these questions, take these steps:

1. Self-monitor. Keep a separate diary for a week to assess just what you are eating and how you are exercising in terms of timing and balance—and portions! Even look at your water intake: Dehydration will force the body to retain fluids. Drink up!

2. Don't assume that the scale is always a true measure of what is going on with the body. If exercise levels are at adequate levels five to seven days a week, you may be putting on muscle but losing fat, thus losing inches even if you are not losing pounds. It is always a good idea to do several body measurements to have a second objective way to monitor progress.

3. What else is going on in your life? Is the stress level too high and energy draining? Do you let that stress undermine your self-image, commitment, energy, and self-worth?

4. Put variety into your eating and your exercise! Our bodies really do adjust to a level of fitness and caloric energy—even to the same kinds of food day after day. Here is where an endurance activity such as a 1½- to two-hour walk or hike on the weekend can start weight loss again. The best programs for weight and fat loss emphasize safe, injury-free techniques, endurance or longer distances, and increased frequency (five to seven days is best) or increased intensity. Interval training works well here. An example would be to walk for ten minutes, racewalk or jog for twelve steps, walk, and alternate per your fitness tolerance to build stamina and increase caloric expenditure. Other techniques include finding simple ways to add short bouts of activity throughout the day. Try walking hills and/or using walking poles to increase your metabolic burn. Add a ten- to twenty-minute walk or bike-ride after dinner or use an Exercycle. Take an exercise class such as Spinning or Pilates to help reduce stress.

There are many ways to get off a plateau, but they take effort, commitment, and balance—and NOT GIVING UP healthy living to take revenge on the scale.

Staying the Course

Remember, The Smart Weigh plan is intended to create a healthier lifestyle—not just shed pounds (though you'll do that, too).

You may be thinking: But this will take too long! I want to be thin *now*! Well, the truth is, it will take longer than a fad diet, but the results will last this time. You won't be fighting the same battles day after day, month after month, year after year. This is a strategy gradually to change the habits and attitudes that may have sabotaged your past efforts. It's not enough to eat healthful foods and exercise for only a few weeks or even several months.

Remember, it's not a diet—it's a new way of living. And that takes thought, planning, and action. Living The Smart Weigh builds a powerful momentum that will support healthy goals for a lifetime. But this momentum will only be maintained through establishing practical strategies for living The Smart Weigh—while traveling, eating out, grocery shopping, and preparing foods at home.

PART 2

REAL-LIFE
STRATEGIES

CHAPTER 9

SMART WEIGH
MEAL PLANS

MY SMART WEIGH MEAL-PLANNING guides give you a detailed strategy for fueling your body with the right foods at the right time. The emphasis is not on just what to eat, but how, when, and how much.

The weight-loss meal plan for women of normal activity provides approximately 1,500 calories a day; the weight-loss meal plan for men and very active women provides approximately 1,800 calories per day; the weight-loss plan for very active men provides 2,200 calories per day. I have also provided tips for boosting your energy quickly.

Portion sizes in each of these plans may need to be adjusted for individual caloric needs. Remember, the number of calories you need depends on your age, size, weight, level of activity, and even stress levels. So don't get caught up in counting every calorie you eat. Instead, focus on eating great foods, prepared in great ways, that will work with your metabolism to release your body's natural ability to burn those calories!

You'll be eating plenty of food at meals, plus two or three snacks,

MEAL-PLANNING TIPS

- **Go for color, go for grains.** Go for blueberries, raspberries, mangoes, papayas, watermelon, honeydew, cantaloupe, apples, oranges, or grapefruit. Go for broccoli, spinach, romaine lettuce, sweet potatoes, and carrots. And vary your breads: try whole-grain English muffins, pita pockets, tortillas, or rolls.
- **Eat beans five or more times a week.** Legumes are one of the highest-fiber foods you can find. Beans are especially high in soluble fiber, which lowers cholesterol levels, and folate, which lowers levels of another risk factor for heart disease, homocysteine. (Quick Tip: To reduce sodium in canned beans by about one-third, rinse off the canning liquid before using. Or look for canned beans with no added sodium.)
- **Have a soy food every day.** This could be soy milk, soy protein isolate powder added to a power shake, soy cheese, tofu, soy nuts, a Boca burger, or tempeh.
- **Eat fish four times a week.** To get the most omega-3s, choose salmon, canned white albacore tuna in water, rainbow trout, anchovies, herring, sardines, and mackerel. Or get a plant version of omega-3 fat in flaxseed and canola oil.
- **Eat nuts five times a week.** Learn to incorporate these luscious morsels into your diet almost every day. The key to eating nuts healthfully is not to eat too many; they're so high in calories that you could easily gain weight. To help avoid temptation, keep nuts in your fridge—where they are safe from oxidizing and turning rancid and where they are out of sight. Sprinkle 2 tablespoons a day on cereal, yogurt, veggies, salads, or wherever the crunch and rich flavor appeal to you.
- Begin adding 1 tablespoon oat bran, 1 tablespoon of wheat bran, and 1 tablespoon of flaxseed to cereal; gradually increase to 2 tablespoons of each.

properly balanced in whole-food simple and complex carbohydrates, proteins, and fats. But if you get really hungry at other times of the day, have a piece of fruit with 1 ounce low-fat or soy cheese or ½ cup skim or soy milk. Drink as much water and seltzer as you like—but definitely get in 64 ounces every day. Limit your intake of caffeinated beverages such as coffee, tea, or soda.

It will take two to three days for your body to stabilize—and for you to feel an increase in energy and to regulate your appetite. In about ten to twelve days, you will notice when your body reminds you that it's time for a power snack or meal—every two to three hours. This is a very good thing—a sign that your body chemistries are stabilizing.

As you familiarize yourself with the meal plans below, refer to the lists of healthy carbs and proteins on pages 43–45 to refresh your memory about your best choices. The power snack choices on page 41 will give you direction in converting the following snack guidelines into a variety of minimeals. I've also provided a Smart Weigh grocery list (pages 162–165) with many specific suggestions of what to bring home from the market so you'll always have handy the makings for healthy meals.

The Smart Weigh Weight-Loss Meal Plan for Women

• Breakfast (within ½ hour of rising)

SIMPLE CARB: 1 serving fresh fruit

COMPLEX CARB: 2 slices whole-wheat toast OR 1 whole-grain English muffin or bagel (may top with 1 teaspoon all-fruit jam, the melted cheese or light cream cheese from protein, or use the optional 1 teaspoon butter) OR 2 homemade whole-grain low-fat muffins OR 1½ cups whole-grain cereal with added bran/flaxseed

PROTEIN: 2 ounces low-fat cheese or ½ cup low-fat cottage/ricotta cheese OR 4 tablespoons light cream cheese OR 2 eggs (three times/week) or 2 egg whites or egg substitute OR 1 cup skim milk or nonfat yogurt for cereal

OPTIONAL FAT: 1 teaspoon butter for toast or muffin OR 1 teaspoon olive or canola oil for cooking OR 1 tablespoon chopped nuts as topping for cereal or yogurt

• Morning Snack (2 to 3 hours after breakfast)

As a whole power snack, may have ¼ cup trail mix (page 125) OR choose a combination of:

SIMPLE CARB: 1 piece of fresh fruit

PROTEIN: 2 ounces part-skim or soy cheese OR 1 cup nonfat yogurt OR 8 ounces skim or soy milk OR ½ cup low-fat cottage/ricotta cheese

• Lunch (2 to 3 hours after morning snack)

SIMPLE CARB: Begin your meal with 1 piece fruit OR 1 cup cooked vegetables OR 1 cup low-fat vegetable soup

COMPLEX CARB: 1 slice whole-grain bread OR 1 baked potato OR ½ whole-wheat pita OR 1 whole-wheat tortilla OR ½ cup brown rice or whole-grain pasta

PROTEIN: 3 ounces cooked poultry, fish, seafood, lean beef, or low-fat cheese OR ¾ cup cooked legumes

HEALTHY MUNCHIES: Raw vegetables as desired (up to 2 cups) with lemon juice, vinegar, mustard, salsa, or no-oil salad dressing

OPTIONAL FAT: May use 1 tablespoon salad dressing OR 1 teaspoon olive or canola oil to make your own salad dressing or to cook with OR 1 teaspoon butter for bread or potato OR 2 tablespoons sour cream on potato OR 1 tablespoon light mayonnaise on a sandwich OR 1 tablespoon chopped nuts sprinkled on foods

• Afternoon Snack (2 to 3 hours after lunch)

COMPLEX CARB: 5 whole-grain crackers OR ½ whole-wheat pita OR 1 ounce baked tortilla chips (with salsa, if desired) OR 1 slice whole-wheat bread OR 1 whole-wheat tortilla

PROTEIN: 1 ounce part-skim or fat-free cheese OR 1 ounce lean meat OR ⅓ cup low-fat bean dip (with chips above or wrapped in tortilla) OR ½ cup nonfat yogurt OR ¼ cup low-fat cottage/ricotta cheese

• Dinner (2 to 3 hours after afternoon snack)

SIMPLE CARB: Begin with 1 piece of fruit or ½ cup mixed fruit OR 1 cup low-fat vegetable soup AND then enjoy another serving of fruit OR 1 cup nonstarchy vegetables with dinner

COMPLEX CARB: ½ cup cooked brown rice or whole-grain pasta OR ½ cup starchy vegetables OR 1 small baked sweet potato

PROTEIN: 2 to 3 ounces cooked skinless poultry, seafood, fish, lean beef OR ½ cup cooked legumes

HEALTHY MUNCHIES: Raw vegetables (up to 2 cups) as desired with lemon juice, vinegar, salsa, or no-oil salad dressing

OPTIONAL FAT: May use 1 tablespoon salad dressing OR 1 teaspoon olive or canola oil to make your own salad dressing or to cook with OR 1 teaspoon butter for bread or potato OR 2 tablespoons sour cream on potato OR 1 tablespoon light mayonnaise on a sandwich OR 1 tablespoon chopped nuts sprinkled on foods

• Night Snack (at least ½ hour before bedtime)

COMPLEX CARB: ¾ cup whole-grain cereal OR 1 slice whole-grain bread

PROTEIN: ½ cup skim or soy milk or nonfat yogurt (with cereal) OR 1 ounce lean meat OR 1 ounce low-fat or soy cheese (melted atop bread)

The Smart Weigh Weight-Loss Meal Plan for Men and Very Active Women

• Breakfast (within ¹/₂ hour of rising)

SIMPLE CARB: 1 serving fresh fruit

COMPLEX CARB: 2 slices whole-wheat toast OR 1 whole-grain English muffin (may top with 1 teaspoon all-fruit jam, the melted cheese, or light cream cheese from protein, or use the optional 1 teaspoon butter) OR 2 homemade whole-grain low-fat muffins OR 1½ cups whole-grain cereal with added bran/flaxseed

PROTEIN: 2 ounces low-fat cheese or ½ cup low-fat cottage/ricotta cheese OR 4 tablespoons light cream cheese OR 2 eggs (three times a week) or 2 egg whites or egg substitute OR 1 cup skim milk or nonfat yogurt for cereal

OPTIONAL FAT: 1 teaspoon butter for toast or muffin OR 1 teaspoon olive or canola oil for cooking OR 1 tablespoon chopped nuts as topping for cereal or yogurt

• Morning Snack (2 to 3 hours after breakfast)

As a whole power snack, may have ½ cup trail mix (page 125) OR choose a combination of:

SIMPLE CARB: 1 piece of fruit

Complex Carb: 5 whole-grain crackers OR ½ whole-wheat pita OR 1 ounce baked tortilla chips (with salsa, if desired) OR 1 slice whole-wheat bread OR 1 whole-wheat tortilla OR 2 pieces whole-grain Crispbread

PROTEIN: 2 ounces part-skim or soy cheese OR 2 ounces lean meat OR 1 cup nonfat yogurt OR ½ cup low-fat cottage/ricotta cheese

• Lunch (2 to 3 hours after midmorning snack)

SIMPLE CARB: Begin your meal with 1 piece of fruit or low-fat vegetable soup AND then enjoy another serving of fruit OR 1 cup cooked vegetables with your lunch

COMPLEX CARB: 2 slices whole-grain bread OR 1 baked potato OR 1 whole-wheat pita/tortilla OR 1 cup brown rice or whole-grain pasta

PROTEIN: 3 ounces cooked poultry, fish, seafood, lean beef, or low-fat cheese OR 1 cup cooked legumes

HEALTHY MUNCHIES: Raw vegetables as desired (up to 2 cups) with lemon juice, vinegar, mustard, salsa, or no-oil salad dressing

OPTIONAL FAT: May use 1 tablespoon salad dressing OR 1 teaspoon olive or canola oil to make your own salad dressing or to cook with OR 1 teaspoon butter for bread or potato OR 2 tablespoons sour cream for potato OR 1 tablespoon light mayonnaise on a sandwich OR 1 tablespoon chopped nuts sprinkled on foods

• Afternoon Snack (2 to 3 hours after lunch)

SIMPLE CARB: 1 piece of fruit

COMPLEX CARB: 5 whole-grain crackers OR ½ whole-wheat pita OR 1 ounce baked tortilla chips (with salsa, if desired) OR 1 slice whole-wheat bread OR 1 whole-wheat tortilla OR 2 pieces whole-grain Crispbread

PROTEIN: 2 ounces part-skim or soy cheese OR 2 ounces lean meat OR ⅔ cup low-fat bean dip (with chips above or wrapped in tortilla) OR 1 cup nonfat yogurt OR ½ cup low-fat cottage/ricotta cheese

• Dinner (2 to 3 hours after afternoon snack)

SIMPLE CARB: Begin with 1 piece of fruit or ½ cup mixed fruit OR 1 cup low-fat vegetable soup AND then enjoy another serving of fruit OR 1 cup nonstarchy vegetables with dinner

COMPLEX CARB: 1 cup brown rice or whole-grain pasta OR 1 cup starchy vegetables OR 1 baked sweet potato

PROTEIN: 3 ounces cooked skinless poultry, seafood, fish, lean beef OR ¾ cup cooked legumes

HEALTHY MUNCHIES: Raw vegetables as desired (up to 2 cups) with lemon juice, vinegar, mustard, salsa, or no-oil salad dressing

OPTIONAL FAT: May use 1 tablespoon salad dressing OR 1 teaspoon olive or canola oil to make your own salad dressing or to cook with OR 1 teaspoon butter for bread or potato OR 2 tablespoons sour cream for potato OR 1 tablespoon light mayonnaise on a sandwich OR 1 tablespoon chopped nuts sprinkled on foods

• Night Snack (at least ½ hour before bedtime)

COMPLEX CARB: ¾ cup whole-grain cereal or 1 slice whole-grain bread

PROTEIN: 1 cup skim or soy milk or nonfat yogurt (with cereal) OR 2 ounces lean meat OR 2 ounces low-fat or soy cheese (melted atop bread)

The Smart Weight-Loss Meal Plan for Very Active Men

• Breakfast (within ¹/₂ hour of rising)

SIMPLE CARB: 2 servings fresh fruit

COMPLEX CARB: 2 slices whole-wheat toast OR 1 whole-grain English muffin (may top with 1 teaspoon all-fruit jam, the melted cheese, or light cream cheese from protein, or use the optional 2 teaspoons butter) OR 2 homemade whole-grain low-fat muffins OR 1½ cups whole-grain cereal with added bran/flaxseed

PROTEIN: 3 ounces low-fat cheese or ¾ cup low-fat cottage/ricotta cheese OR 6 tablespoons light cream cheese OR 3 whole eggs (times a week) or 3 egg whites or ¾ cup egg substitute OR 1½ cups skim milk or nonfat yogurt for cereal

OPTIONAL FAT: 2 teaspoons butter for toast or muffin OR 2 teaspoons olive or canola oil for cooking OR 2 tablespoons chopped nuts as topping for cereal or yogurt

• Morning Snack (2 to 3 hours after breakfast)

As a whole power snack, may have ½ cup trail mix (page 125) OR choose a combination of:

SIMPLE CARB: 1 piece of fruit

COMPLEX CARB: 5 whole-grain crackers OR ½ whole-wheat pita OR 1 ounce baked tortilla chips (with salsa, if desired) OR 1 slice whole-wheat bread OR 1 whole-wheat tortilla OR 2 pieces whole-grain Crispbread

PROTEIN: 2 ounces part-skim or soy cheese OR 2 ounces lean meat OR ⅔ cup low-fat bean dip (with chips above or wrapped in tortilla) OR 1 cup nonfat yogurt OR ½ cup low-fat cottage/ricotta cheese

• Lunch (2 to 3 hours after morning snack)

SIMPLE CARB: Begin your meal with 1 piece fruit or low-fat vegetable soup AND then enjoy another serving fruit OR 1 cup cooked vegetables with your lunch

COMPLEX CARB: 2 slices whole-grain bread OR 1 baked potato OR
   1 whole-wheat pita/tortilla OR 1 cup brown rice/whole-grain pasta

PROTEIN: 4 ounces cooked poultry, fish, seafood, lean beef, or low-fat
   cheese OR 1 cup cooked legumes

HEALTHY MUNCHIES: Raw vegetables as desired (up to 2 cups) with lemon
   juice, vinegar, mustard, or no-oil salad dressing

OPTIONAL FAT: May use 2 tablespoons salad dressing OR 2 teaspoons
   olive or canola oil to make your own salad dressing or to cook with
   OR 2 teaspoons butter for bread or potato OR 4 tablespoons sour
   cream for potato OR 2 tablespoons light mayonnaise on a sandwich
   OR 2 tablespoons chopped nuts sprinkled on foods

• Afternoon Snack (2 to 3 hours after lunch)

Repeat earlier snack choices

• Dinner (2 to 3 hours after afternoon snack)

SIMPLE CARB: Begin with 1 piece of fruit or ½ cup mixed fruit OR 1 cup
   low-fat vegetable soup AND then enjoy another serving of fruit and
   1 cup nonstarchy vegetables with dinner

COMPLEX CARB: 1½ cups brown rice or whole-grain pasta OR 1½ cups
   starchy vegetables OR 1 baked sweet potato

PROTEIN: 4 ounces cooked skinless poultry, seafood, fish, lean beef OR
   1 cup cooked legumes

HEALTHY MUNCHIES: Raw vegetables (up to 2 cups) as desired with lemon
   juice, vinegar, or no-oil salad dressing

OPTIONAL FAT: May use 2 tablespoons salad dressing OR 2 teaspoons
   olive or canola oil to make your own salad dressing or to cook with
   OR 2 teaspoons butter for bread or potato OR 4 tablespoons sour
   cream for potato OR 2 tablespoons light mayonnaise on a sandwich
   OR 2 tablespoons chopped nuts sprinkled on foods

• Night Snack (at least ½ hour before bedtime)

SIMPLE CARB: 1 piece of fruit

COMPLEX CARB: ¾ cup whole-grain cereal or 1 slice whole-grain bread

PROTEIN: 1½ cups skim or soy milk or non-fat yogurt (with cereal) OR 2
   ounces lean meat OR 2 ounces low-fat or soy cheese (melted atop bread)

Boost Your Energy the Smart Weigh

If you are in need of immediate energy, working to stabilize your blood sugars because of hypoglycemia (or just trying to break the sugar habit), trying to overcome gastric distress (even morning sickness), or dealing with high stress levels, follow your appropriate meal plan with these adjustments:

- Have 4 to 6 ounces unsweetened juice (if citrus is "hard" on your stomach first thing in the morning, try "soft" juices like unsweetened apple or white grape juice) immediately on rising; follow with breakfast within the next half-hour.
- Add in an extra power snack (see page 41) both morning and afternoon so that you are eating more often—every two hours. Adjust the timing based on your day's schedule (if you are up earlier or later). Follow this plan for two to three days—up to three weeks is advised. By then, you may be energized enough to maintain the basic Smart Weigh meal plan that's right for you.
- Drink more water, but after meals and snacks rather than on an empty stomach.
- Always have your meal's simple carbohydrate at the beginning of the meal or snack to get the quicker energy release that it provides.

What About Sweets?

A heavy sugar intake brings a pleasurable rise in feel-good brain chemicals that will be followed by a quick fall a few hours later. That dip often triggers "eating for a lift" to relieve the fatigue, brain fog, and mood drop. Usually the chosen food is again high in sugar, and the seesaw effect continues. Then the guilt tapes begin to play: You've already blown it, so go ahead and finish the cookies before you get "back" to healthy eating. And the more you eat, the more you crave, trying to get that same boost.

Equalizing your brain chemistries is a key to living The Smart Weigh because too-low levels of serotonin and endorphins trigger the

WHAT ABOUT POWER BARS AND ENERGY SHAKES?

The question is, are nutritional bars and canned shakes the nutrition panacea they are touted to be? Well... they are certainly better choices than downing a cola and fries and calling it lunch, but they are a much worse choice than a grilled chicken salad. Better than no lunch at all—but not better than the real McCoy. A can a day won't keep the doctor away!

The problem with manufactured nutrition in a can—or a bar—is that they simply can't duplicate naturally the collection of nutrients in real food. They lack adequate fiber and valuable phytochemicals such as isoflavones, carotenoids, and other plant-derived compounds that get you well and keep you well. Even fruit and dairy-based shakes don't comprise a whole healthy diet—but they can be great as a snack or part of a meal.

And it's not just about nutrient needs—it's also about pleasure. When people turn to liquid lunches or a bar, they deprive themselves of the pleasure of real food, with all its varied textures and smells. In addition, although an energy bar or shake may provide the calories of a chicken sandwich, a bowl of strawberries, and a glass of milk, you're not getting any of the nutrients naturally found in those foods. And that's the long-term problem when these energy bars become chronic substitutes for meals or when eaten in large quantities.

The average person, even the moderately active one, doesn't need energy to come from an engineered bar—he or she simply needs to eat, and to eat often and well. Yet, the "energy" term is very seductive; people feel they're getting more than they are. What you get from one of these bars is really calories, but the term "calorie bar" wouldn't gross the same sales!

Still, if push comes to shove, and the choice is an energy bar over a candy bar, or no meal at all, then choose those that have about 220 to 250 calories, less than 2 grams of fat per 100 calories, over 10 grams of protein, and about 45 to 50 grams of carbohydrate—a snack for a would be weight-gainer, a meal for a would be weight- loser or maintainer. Just be sure to get real food at the next stop.

craving for a drug that will provide fuel for these neurotransmitters. And there is evidence that some people use sweet foods and refined carbohydrates as powerful mood-altering drugs, and experience the similar roller-coaster of behavior and thoughts of an addict.

If you're serious about losing weight, cutting back on sugar is essential. The average American consumes a whopping nineteen teaspoons, or 304 calories, of sugar added to foods each day. That includes sugars added by manufacturers to foods like soda, flavored yogurts, and cookies—as well as those added directly by the consumer, such as to iced tea or cereals. The amount of weight you'll lose in one year if you cut that added sugar in half? Sixteen pounds for an average adult.

If sugar is affecting your well-being, make it your goal to cut back on your daily use of sweets and other refined carbs and eat whole carbohydrates and fruits to stabilize your body chemistries and satisfy your natural craving for sugar. Sweets are not worth robbing yourself of your precious energy and stamina.

The Smart Weigh meal plan is designed to load every calorie with life-enhancing nutrition. High-sugar foods bring you lots of empty calories and little else. People who avoid all sugar for a month or two often find that they lose their craving for it. It's worth trying!

But remember not to make any food absolutely forbidden. That could just set you up for a binge on what you "can't" have.

What About Salt?

Although salt is certainly not the number one nutritional evil, it is a concern. The main problem is the amount we use—way, way too much. The average American consumes more than eight times his or her daily requirement—about fifteen pounds per year. This is the equivalent of two to four teaspoons of salt each day. Hypertension, fluid retention, and kidney dysfunction are just a few of the health problems to which those little white granules contribute.

In America today, approximately sixty million people have abnormally high blood pressure, and two million more are adding to the ranks each year. This means that one out of five people are predisposed to high blood pressure—and salt's impact. However, it's not possible to identify who is at risk, so it's wise to practice prevention and cut back on excess salt—even before a doctor tells you that you must.

Salt is made up of 60 percent sodium and 40 percent chloride. In the human body, excess sodium becomes a troublemaker, creating a temporary buildup of fluids, making it harder for the heart to pump blood through the system, and causing a rise in the blood pressure (hypertension). Other factors besides salt intake, such as heredity, a low intake of fruits and vegetables, a high saturated fat intake, and obesity, can also contribute to hypertension.

Unlike heredity, salt consumption is a factor within our control; unfortunately, for the majority of Americans, it is out of control. Shaking the salt habit can be difficult because salt plays a big part in the enjoyment of food. It serves as a catalyst for flavor, enhancing the taste of other ingredients. The key to making this good-for-you cut-back is to learn to prepare foods in ways that naturally enhance flavor so less salt is needed for good taste. You'll notice that many of The Smart Weigh recipes use herbs and spices, which allows you to drastically reduce the amount of salt.

What About Alcohol?

You may have watched it on *60 Minutes*; you may have read about it in the newspaper. It's called "The French Paradox," and it's all about wine, particularly red wine, being good for you. You read that a moderate amount of alcohol, in any form, actually extends life, and may help to offset the negative health effects of a high-fat diet. Your friend's cardiologist recommended that she drink a glass of Merlot every night to raise her HDL cholesterol; it would be good for her. But is it true? And, if so, how does that advice fit into The Smart Weigh meal plan?

It is true that a moderate intake of alcohol has been found to have some positive health benefits, and the research is strong and promising enough that many physicians actually recommend a glass of wine to their patients. But also true is that, over time, excessive alcohol can result in a chronic energy drain; its impact on blood sugars increases appetite, interrupts sleep, and interferes with nutrient absorption. The extra calories it adds to your diet can contribute to weight gain or prevent weight loss. And more than moderate intake can damage your internal organs (such as your liver, intestines, and heart) and increase risk of cancer, particularly liver and breast cancer.

The fact is, the medical benefits of wine or other spirits are just not compelling enough to encourage people who don't drink to begin. The U.S. dietary guidelines say this: "If you drink, do so in moderation." But what is moderation? It's considered to be a four- to six-ounce glass of wine, one light beer, or one and a half ounces of hard liquor a day. Because of the impact of alcohol on your blood sugars, it's best to fit it into The Smart Weigh meal plan as a simple carbohydrate, substituting it for one of your pieces of fruit at a meal, or how about a refreshing mineral water with lime instead?

Great and Great for You!

For food to be enjoyable, it needs to taste great; if it doesn't taste good, it has limited power to satisfy. But let's face it: Time is short. On weeknights, especially, spending less time in the kitchen becomes a clear necessity if we are to spend more time enjoying our food, friends, and family, in addition to some quiet time for personal recharge. But too often, in our catch-as-catch-can way of doing things, something is compromised: taste, health, or the entire satis-faction of making and enjoying a home-cooked meal. Yet many interesting and delicious meals can be made in short order.

Most cooks spend sixteen to forty-five minutes preparing dinner, according to a recent survey by market research firm The NPD Group. Small wonder that there's a boomlet in convenience foods, recipes that rely on pantry staples, and cookbooks and magazines promising to cut kitchen time. Studies show that people want to make a contribution to the meal they've made their families, but they don't necessarily want to make the whole thing.

That's where convenience products come in that call for minimal kitchen work, such as chopping fresh herbs for a rice mix or adding chicken strips to a frozen pasta-and-vegetable entrée. Most people don't really hate to cook; what they hate is the stress and spending more time in the kitchen. They hate having to clean up more mess and to feel overwhelmed.

But it needn't be so! The key to great foods that are great for you is being equipped with a well-stocked kitchen and the knowledge of how to put together quick and easy meals. Learn to shop and cook meals The Smart Weigh.

CHAPTER 10

SMART WEIGH SHOPPING GUIDE AND RECIPES

HEALTHY HOME COOKING IS still possible—even in the express lane. Keeping a well-stocked pantry, planning a week's worth of healthy menus, and knowing some shortcuts can simplify weekday meal preparation enough to make it, if not a joy, at least less of a hassle. Healthy home cooking is cheaper, and you can control the calories and fat a lot better. With that said, here are some suggestions to beat the last-minute dinnertime blues and to put together meals that are destined to satisfy the taste buds and the time-budget:

- Set aside fifteen minutes a week with your family to plan dinners. After a couple of weeks, you'll have menus that you can use over and over.
- Streamline shopping. With a week's worth of menus in hand, it's easy to cut back on last-minute trips to the store. Choosing recipes with fewer ingredients will speed you through the checkout lane.
- Use the supermarket salad bar for diced or cubed fresh veggies— you buy exactly the amount you need. Also stock up on bags of

precut salad greens from the produce section. They're dated for freshness, so go for the latest date possible.

- Get peeled, freshly cooked shrimp at the shrimp counter, grilled chicken breasts from the deli. Instead of cooking turkey breast, buy eight ounces of unsliced cooked turkey breast, then dice at home.
- Keep your cupboards well stocked and organized. Besides canned broth, canned tomatoes, and whole-grain pastas, have a few nonperishables on hand to add interest to those basics: chutneys, dried mushrooms, flavored vinegars, etc. It's time-savvy to group similar items together and always restock in the same way. Knowing what's on hand saves rummaging through cabinets when cooking and making shopping lists.

The Well-Stocked Kitchen

Take a long look at what typically is in your grocery cart. If it's a grease and sugar trap loaded with butter, bacon, and Twinkies, chances are you're not going to be producing slim fixings on the home front. A well-stocked kitchen makes the difference between efficiently putting together healthy flavorful foods and a meal-time-blues headache or a fast-food nightmare. Now is a good time to strengthen and streamline your grocery shopping, your fridge, and, thereby, your body.

Here are some guidelines for adding the health advantage to your shopping cart—and your Smart Weigh grocery list to be sure you bring home "the right stuff:"

Choose Cereals and Breads: Whole grain is a must for fiber and nutrition. The word "whole" should be the first word of the ingredient list, such as "whole wheat," and "whole oats." Also check labels for hidden fats and sugars; some cereals, like granola, are nutritional nightmares in a bowl. Cereals should have fewer than five grams of added sugar, excluding any from dried fruit they may contain. Also, your natural foods store is likely to carry a variety of 100 percent whole-wheat products, including whole-grain English muffins, bagels, tortillas, pitas, and crackers.

Buy the Basics: Stock up on whole-wheat or artichoke pastas and brown rice. Incorporate barley, oats, cracked wheat, and cornmeal into recipes. Include dried or canned beans, split peas, lentils, and chickpeas.

Fend Against Fats and Oils: Don't use polyunsaturated oils, but instead use olive or canola oil in small amounts. Select reduced-fat or light mayonnaise rather than the fat-free (chemical-filled) varieties. Avoid hydrogenated fats whenever possible—label-reading is a must here.

Pick Produce: For the best produce, choose what is in season—a good price and an abundant supply will tell you a fruit or vegetable is at its peak. Ask at your grocery store or farmer's market which are the freshest buying days and where the produce is grown; search for locally grown and in-season fruits and vegetables. Out-of-season produce is more expensive and often imported. If it's imported, it may be only spot-checked for pesticide residues. When fresh is not possible, frozen is the next best choice—but avoid vegetables prepared with butters or sauces, or fruits packed with sugar. Freezing foods doesn't destroy their nutrients and quality as readily as canning does.

WHEN BIGGER ISN'T BETTER!

The next time you add that economy-sized box of cornflakes to your shopping cart, think twice. A recent University of Illinois study asked women to take enough spaghetti from a box to make dinner for two—no measuring allowed. When the women were given a standard one-pound box, they grabbed an average of 234 strands of pasta, enough to make two 350-calorie servings. Not bad. Yet, when they were given a two-pound box, they averaged 302 strands—a 29 percent increase, and a whopping 102-calorie difference per serving.

Researchers got the same result with cooking oil. The women poured 192 more calories' worth into a pan when they used a 32-ounce bottle as opposed to a 16-ounce bottle.

The lesson? If you're buying the family pack, be sure to measure!

Shopping The Smart Weigh

I advocate "real foods" rather than highly processed packaged food. For example, real orange juice or frozen concentrate is far superior to fortified orange-flavored drink. Think "Mother Nature" when you shop. You don't have to shop at a health food store to get healthful foods; your grocery store is crammed full of them.

Follow these "trim the fat" tips when you're ready to shop for, plan for, and prepare food that looks great, tastes great, and is great for you:

- Switch from whole-milk dairy products to skim or 1 percent milk, buttermilk, and nonfat plain yogurt. Look for fat-free or lower fat versions of favorite cheeses such as ricotta, pot, or farmers cheese; skim-milk mozzarella; cottage cheese; and fat-free or "light" cream cheese. Check the label to be sure they have less than five grams of fat per ounce. You may also want to try some of the new soy food versions of dairy. You'll get more than you're bargaining for—they are loaded with substances that bless you with disease protection.

- At the deli, go for the leanest cuts. Select sliced turkey or chicken, lean ham, and low-fat cheeses instead of the usual "lunch meats." Limit use of high-fat, high-sodium, processed sausages and meats, hot dogs, bacon, and salami.

- Use this formula to figure the fat percentage of calories when assessing whether food products are as good as they claim: nine calories per gram of fat, times grams of fat, divided by calories per serving. Buy foods that derive less than 25 percent of their calories from fat.

- Buy whole-grain and freshly baked breads and rolls. They have more flavor and do not need butter or margarine to taste good.

- Use the new all-fruit jams on breads or toast, rather than fat spreads like butter or margarine.

- Keep an abundant supply of fresh fruits and cut, munchy vegetables on hand for snacking. Buy light popcorn, breads, and low-fat crackers rather than chips and cookies. Substitute sorbet or frozen juice bars for ice cream.

Once your pantry and fridge are stocked with the "right stuff," you're equipped to put together meals in short order. These tips will help to streamline your time in the kitchen.

- Use your freezer as a pantry as well. If you're grilling two chicken breasts, why not grill twelve and store ten? Besides storing defrost-and-serve meals and leftovers, use the freezer for quick-to-thaw meal makers such as frozen veggies, extra cooked brown rice, and freezer-to-oven proteins, such as your advanced grilled chicken or meats.

- Work on more than one recipe at a time. People tend to do one recipe, finish it, and go on to the next. And that just takes too much time. Whatever takes longest, do first. That way, the rest of the meal prep falls into place at the right time.

- Use speedier cooking methods. Forget roasting or braising and go with broiling, sautéeing, or steaming. And try pressure cooking—particularly for preparing whole grains. It can cut cooking time by a third.

- Invest in good sharp knives. You may not even need to haul out the food processor or chopper.

- Quick-thaw with your microwave. Stick frozen chicken breasts in the microwave on defrost, cook them at full power for two to three minutes, then slice the still partially frozen chicken into strips. Throw them into a skillet—they will be thin enough to heat through quickly.

- Cut down on cleanup. Try to keep the number of utensils to a minimum and use nonstick pans whenever possible. And my best tip: Get someone else to wash the dishes!

- Designate a fall-back recipe. Find one recipe you love and tape it into your cupboard door nearest your stove. Keep the ingredients for the recipe on hand at all times. You'll make it when time is crunched to the max. My favorite quick meal is Baked Spaghetti. (See recipe on page 173.)

continued on page 166

THE SMART WEIGH GROCERY LIST

GRAINS AND BREADS
❑ Barley

Brown rice:
❑ Instant
❑ Long-grain
❑ Basmati
❑ Wild rice

❑ Buck wheat
❑ Bulgar
❑ Cornmeal
❑ Couscous

Tortillas, flour:
❑ Mission
❑ Buena Vida fat-free

❑ whole-wheat bagels
❑ 100% whole-wheat bread *("whole" is the first word of the ingredients)*
❑ whole-wheat English muffins
❑ whole-wheat hamburger buns

Whole-wheat or artichoke pasta:
❑ Angel hair
❑ Elbows
❑ Flat
❑ Lasagna
❑ Orzo
❑ Penne
❑ Spaghetti
❑ Rotini (spirals)
❑ whole-wheat pastry flour

❑ whole-wheat pita bread

CEREALS
(whole grain and less than 5 grams of added sugar excluding dried fruit)
❑ All Bran With Extra Fiber
❑ Cheerios
❑ Familia Müesli
❑ Bran Buds with psyllium
❑ Grape-Nuts
❑ Grits
❑ Kashi GoLEAN Crunch!
❑ Kellogg's Just Right
❑ Kellogg's Low-Fat Granola
❑ Kellogg's Nutri-Grain Almond Raisin
❑ Kellogg's Raisin Mini-Wheats
❑ Kellogg's Special K
❑ Nabisco Shredded Wheat
❑ Ralston Müesli
❑ Post Bran Flakes
❑ Shredded Wheat 'N Bran
❑ Wheatena

Oats:
❑ Old-fashioned
❑ Quick-cooking

Unprocessed bran:
❑ Oat

❑ Wheat
❑ Rice

CRACKERS

Crispbread:
❑ Kavli
❑ Wasa
❑ Crispy cakes
❑ Health Valley graham crackers
❑ Harvest Crisps 5-Grain *(not all whole grain, but good for variety)*
❑ Ryvita Wholegrain crispbread
❑ Ry Krisp

DAIRY
❑ Butter
❑ Light butter

Cheese *(low-fat—fewer than 5 grams of fat per ounce)*

Cheddar:
❑ Kraft Fat-Free
❑ Kraft Natural Reduced Fat

❑ Cottage cheese *(1% or nonfat)*

Cream cheese:
❑ Philadelphia Light (tub)
❑ Philadelphia Free
❑ Farmer's

❏ Jarlsberg Lite

Mozzarella:
❏ Nonfat
❏ Part-skim
❏ String cheese

Soy Cheese:
❏ Veggie Slices

Nonrefrigerated:
❏ Laughing Cow Light
❏ Parmesan

Ricotta:
❏ Nonfat
❏ Skim milk

❏ Sun-Ni Armenian String
❏ Egg substitute
❏ Eggs
❏ Egg whites
❏ Milk (skim or 1%)
❏ Reduced fat sour cream
❏ Nonfat plain yogurt
❏ Stonyfield Farm yogurt

CANNED GOODS

Chicken broth:
❏ Swanson's
❏ Natural Goodness

❏ Evaporated skim milk

❏ Hearts of Palm

Soups:
❏ Healthy Choice
❏ Pritikin

❏ Progresso:
❏ Hearty Black Bean
❏ Lentil
❏ 99% Fat-Free Chicken Noodle

Tomatoes:
❏ Paste
❏ Sauce
❏ Stewed
❏ Whole
❏ Fresh Cut

CONDIMENTS
❏ Honey

Hot pepper sauce:
❏ Pickapeppa sauce
❏ Shriracha Chili Sauce
❏ Jamaican Hell Fire
❏ Tabasco

Mayonnaise:
❏ Light
❏ Miracle Whip Light

Mustard:
❏ Dijon
❏ Spicy hot

❏ Pepperoncini peppers

Salad dressing:
❏ Bernstein's Reduced Calorie
❏ Good Seasons
❏ Kraft Free
❏ Jardine's fat-free Garlic
❏ Vinaigrette
❏ Pritikin

❏ Soy sauce *(low sodium)*

❏ Salsa or picante sauce

SPICES AND HERBS
❏ Allspice
❏ Basil
❏ Black pepper
❏ Cayenne
❏ Celery seed
❏ Chili powder
❏ Cinnamon
❏ Creole seasoning
❏ Curry
❏ Dill weed
❏ Five spice
❏ Garlic powder
❏ Ginger
❏ Mrs. Dash Original Blend
❏ Mrs. Dash Garlic and Herb Seasoning
❏ Mustard
❏ Nutmeg
❏ Oregano
❏ Onion powder
❏ Paprika
❏ Parsley
❏ Pepper, cracked
❏ Rosemary
❏ Saffron
❏ Salt
❏ Thyme

Fresh herbs:
❏ Basil
❏ Chives
❏ Cilantro
❏ Ginger

continued on page 164

THE SMART WEIGH GROCERY LIST—CONTINUED

❑ Parsley
❑ Rosemary
❑ Thyme

❑ Vanilla extract

❑ Lea & Perrins Worcestershire for Chicken

Vinegars:
❑ Balsamic
❑ Cider
❑ Red wine
❑ Rice wine
❑ Tarragon
❑ White wine

FRUITS
Fresh fruits:
❑ Apples
❑ Apricots
❑ Bananas
❑ Berries
❑ Cherries
❑ Dates *(unsweetened, pitted)*
❑ Grapefruit
❑ Grapes
❑ Kiwi
❑ Lemons
❑ Limes
❑ Mango
❑ Melon
❑ Nectarines
❑ Oranges
❑ Papaya
❑ Peaches

❑ Pears
❑ Pineapple
❑ Plantains
❑ Plums

Dried fruits:
❑ Apricots
❑ Peaches
❑ Pineapple
❑ Raisins *(dark and golden)*
❑ Mixed

VEGETABLES
❑ Asparagus
❑ Beets
❑ Bell peppers
❑ Broccoli
❑ Brussels sprouts
❑ Cabbage
❑ Carrots
❑ Cauliflower
❑ Celery
❑ Corn
❑ Cucumbers
❑ Eggplant
❑ Green beans
❑ Greens
❑ Hot peppers
❑ Kale
❑ Mushrooms
❑ Okra
❑ Onions
❑ Peas
❑ Red Potatoes

❑ Radicchio
❑ Romaine lettuce
❑ Salad greens
❑ Shallots
❑ Simply Potatoes hash browns
❑ Spinach
❑ Squash *(yellow, crookneck)*
❑ Sugar snap peas *(frozen)*
❑ Sun-dried tomatoes
❑ Sweet potatoes
❑ Tomatoes
❑ Whole potatoes
❑ Zucchini

BEANS AND MEATS
Beans and peas:
❑ Black
❑ Chickpeas/ garbanzo beans
❑ Cannelini
❑ Kidney
❑ Lentils
❑ Navy
❑ Pinto
❑ Split peas

❑ Garden Burger

Beef (lean):
❑ Deli-sliced
❑ Ground round
❑ London broil
❑ Round steak

Fish and seafood:
- ❑ Clams
- ❑ Cod
- ❑ Grouper
- ❑ Mussels
- ❑ Salmon
- ❑ Scallops
- ❑ Shrimp
- ❑ Snapper
- ❑ Swordfish
- ❑ Tuna

Lamb:
- ❑ Leg
- ❑ Loin chops

Pork:
- ❑ Canadian bacon
- ❑ Center cut chops
- ❑ Tenderloin

Chicken:
- ❑ Boneless breasts
- ❑ Legs/thighs
- ❑ Whole fryer

Turkey:
- ❑ Bacon
- ❑ Breast
- ❑ Ground, extra lean
- ❑ Deli-sliced
- ❑ Whole

Veal:
- ❑ Chops
- ❑ Cutlets
- ❑ Ground

Water-packed cans:
- ❑ Chicken

- ❑ Salmon
- ❑ Tuna
- ❑ Charlie's Lunch Kit

Soy:
- ❑ Tofu
- ❑ Silk *(milk)*
- ❑ Boca Burgers
- ❑ Tempeh

MISCELLANEOUS
All-fruit spreads and pourable fruit:
- ❑ Knudsen
- ❑ Polaner
- ❑ Smucker's Simply Fruit
- ❑ Welch's Totally Fruit

- ❑ Baking powder
- ❑ Baking soda

Bean dips:
- ❑ Jardine's
- ❑ Guiltless Gourmet

- ❑ Bread crumbs

Cooking oils:
- ❑ Canola
- ❑ Olive
- ❑ Nonstick cooking spray

- ❑ Cornstarch

Fruit Juices *(unsweetened)*
- ❑ Apple
- ❑ Cranberry-apple
- ❑ White grape
- ❑ Orange

Nuts/seeds
(dry-roasted, unsalted):
- ❑ Flaxseed
- ❑ Peanuts
- ❑ Sunflower kernels
- ❑ Pecans
- ❑ Pumpkin seeds
- ❑ Walnuts

Pasta sauce:
- ❑ Pritikin
- ❑ Classico Tomato and Basil
- ❑ Ragú Chunky Gardenstyle

- ❑ Peanut butter *(natural)*

Popcorn:
- ❑ Orville Redenbacher's Natural
- ❑ Light or Smart Pop microwave popcorn
- ❑ Plain kernels

Tortilla chips:
- ❑ Baked Tostitos
- ❑ Guiltless Gourmet

- ❑ Water *(spring or sparkling)*

Wine:
- ❑ Nonalcoholic
- ❑ Red
- ❑ White

When you're planning meals and cooking The Smart Weigh, remember to pay attention to added fat in preparation. Follow these tips for trimming the fat from your diet:

- Eat more fish and skinless poultry, and fewer red meats. If you eat red meats, buy lean and trim well (before and after cooking)—and cook them in a way that diminishes fat, such as grilling, broiling, or roasting on a rack.

- Use marinades, flavored vinegars, plain yogurt, or juices when grilling or broiling to tenderize leaner cuts of meat and seal in their moisture and flavor. Mix these marinades with fresh or dried herbs such as basil, oregano, and parsley to add flavor.

- Limit protein portions to five ounces precooked. After cooking, the size will resemble that of a deck of cards. This is the typical lunch portion of fish or chicken served in a restaurant. (The typical dinner portion is nine ounces.) Let brown rice, whole-grain pastas, potatoes, and vegetables become the centerpiece of your meals.

- Use nonstick cooking sprays and skillets. These will enable you to brown meats without grease and to sauté ingredients in stocks and broths rather than in fats and oils. If a recipe calls for basting a meat in butter or in "its juices," baste instead with tomato, lemon juice, or stocks.

- Skim the fat from soups, stocks, and meat drippings. Refrigerate and remove the hardened surface layer of fat before reheating. As you do, think about that fat hardening in your body, and the great favor you are doing yourself by getting rid of it!

- Use legumes (dried beans and peas) as a main dish. These meat substitutes can be a high-nutrition, low-fat meal. Attempt a switch at least twice each week. If beans have been gaseous in the past, try Beano (available from your pharmacy or health food store); it's a natural enzyme that works wonders for digestion of beans and other gas-forming foods while your body is becoming more tolerant on its own.

- Substitute plain, nonfat yogurt or fat-free ricotta cheese in dips or sauces calling for sour cream or mayonnaise. Also, use these as toppings for baked potatoes and chili. (And don't forget low-fat, flavorful salsa, a great low-cal topping for almost anything.)
- Use two egg whites in place of one whole egg. Egg whites are pure protein; egg yolks are pure fat and cholesterol.

In the pages ahead are suggested menus that incorporate all of my principles for preparing specific dishes and meals The Smart Weigh. Each menu is made up of recipes that have been designed to form a pleasing whole of contrasting flavors, textures, and colors. Each meal is designed with the proper balance of protein, complex carbohydrates, simple carbohydrates, and fat as outlined in The Smart Weigh meal plans in Chapter 9.

The nutrient balance and calorie counts are roughly the same for each breakfast, lunch, and dinner. If you really like one of the meals, or don't care for another, just mix and match meals from one day to the next. A tuna sandwich is fine for breakfast, and an egg-white omelet works just fine for dinner. Substitute green beans if you're not craving asparagus; leave out a spice or herb if you don't have it available. You can also use healthy foods you have on hand to create something new and personally yours.

I have analyzed each recipe for its nutritional value. Besides the calories, carbohydrate, protein, and fat grams, I have included information about sodium and cholesterol for those of you watching these numbers as well. The fat grams are also expressed in terms of the percentage of calories derived from fat in each particular dish. My meals are designed to give less than 25 percent of the calories from fat, with the average dish yielding 17 percent.

Individual recipes that are higher in percentage of fat calories are paired with those having low or no fat to balance the whole meal properly. I have used these profiles to plan balanced meals that give appropriate levels of nutrients. Portion sizes may need to be adjusted to fit caloric needs according to your own individualized meal plan. Don't get caught up in counting every calorie or fat gram—just focus on eating great foods, prepared in great ways, that are great for you.

Most of the recipes in the pages ahead have been my favorites, and many are dishes I've developed for restaurants interested in healthier menu offerings. Many have been passed on to me by friends (often chefs) and family. Some have been developed, others "made over" for The Smart Weigh. There is an endless array of cooking tricks—part art, part science—to turn unhealthy, full-of-fat dishes into tasty, nutritious ones. I have used them all in these recipes, and you may want to use them on some of your favorites as well.

Basically, I use four methods to reduce the amount of fat, calories, and other detrimental substances in a recipe.

- Reduce the amount of high-fat, high-salt ingredients and look for ways to enhance flavor, texture, and nutritive value.
- Replace a high-fat, high-salt ingredient with a different one that is lower in fat and sodium and higher in flavor.
- Use smaller amounts of fattier foods that pack a powerful flavor punch: feta cheese, Parmesan, coconut, toasted nuts, sesame oil, and turkey bacon or sausage made from turkey. I cut the quantity to less than 50 percent of what is called for in the typical recipe.
- Use a cooking method that reduces fat yet enhances moisture and flavor. This reduces or eliminates the need for fats, oils, and rich sauces. Some of the techniques I use most in cooking The Smart Weigh are grilling and broiling, parchment cooking, poaching, sautéing and stir-frying, steaming or boiling, and microwaving.

Getting Started

You'll find that these meals are fresh, fun, and flavorful. They'll fill you with good food and good health. The key is getting started—and remember it's progress, not perfection that counts. You may start with some of the following "grab 'n go" breakfasts. Or you may start packing a more interesting lunch that's healthier and more energizing. It may be one fabulous dinner a week or elements of The Smart Weigh cooking sprinkled throughout all your meals. Wherever you choose to begin—get cooking and have fun!

My Quickest Breakfasts

Don't resort to the food industry's versions of "instant" breakfasts, like toaster fruit pies, granola bars (just candy with oats), and artificially flavored and colored powdered drink mixes. Instead of going for breakfast in the fast lane—and getting much more fat, calories, and sodium than you've bargained for—grab and go with your own quick and easy breakfast:

POWER BREAKFAST SHAKE

½ cup frozen fruit
1 cup skim milk
1 coddled egg white, or ¼ cup egg substitute
2 teaspoons honey
1 teaspoon vanilla
1 tablespoon wheat germ

Blend together until smooth and frothy. You can put all these together in the blender container and place the whole thing in your fridge before bed. In the morning pull it out and place it on the blender apparatus and zap: you've got a drinkable "instant" breakfast that's loaded with whole food nutrients.

Gives 1 complex carbohydrate (wheat germ), 2 ounces protein (milk and egg whites), and 1 simple carbohydrate (fruit).

Serves 1

Per serving: 37 grams carbohydrate; 17 grams protein; 0 grams fat; 0 calories from fat, 2 milligrams cholesterol, 88 milligrams sodium, 216 calories.

SCRAMBLED EGG BURRITO

1 10-inch whole wheat flour tortilla
1 egg, lightly beaten, or $\frac{1}{4}$ cup egg substitute
2 tablespoons (1 ounces) 2-percent milk cheddar or soy cheese, grated
$\frac{1}{4}$ teaspoon creole seasoning (or salt and pepper to taste)
2 tablespoons salsa
$\frac{1}{4}$ cantaloupe, sliced

Heat a nonstick pan or griddle over medium-high heat. Add the tortilla to heat and soften, turning it over after 15 seconds. After another 15 seconds, remove the tortilla from the pan and wrap it in foil to keep warm. Spray the pan with nonstick spray, continuing to heat. Beat together the eggs, grated cheese, and creole seasoning. Add to the pan and scramble. Place the egg mixture on the tortilla and spoon on the salsa. Wrap it up burrito-style. Serve with the sliced cantaloupe. Gives 1 complex carbohydrate (tortilla), 2 ounces protein (eggs and cheese), and 1 simple carbohydrate (cantaloupe).

Serves 1

Per serving: 32 grams carbohydrate; 13 grams protein; 5 grams fat; 20 percent calories from fat (with egg substitute), 8 milligrams cholesterol, 613 milligrams sodium, 223 calories.

HOT OATCAKES WITH BERRIES

4 egg whites
1 cup nonfat ricotta cheese
2 tablespoons canola oil
1 teaspoon vanilla
$\frac{2}{3}$ cup old-fashioned oats, uncooked
$\frac{1}{4}$ teaspoons salt
nonstick cooking spray
4 tablespoons all fruit jam or pourable all-fruit syrup
2 cups mixed berries

Measure the egg whites, ricotta cheese, oil, vanilla, oats, and salt into a blender or food processor and blend for 5 to 6 minutes. Spoon 2 tablespoons batter into a hot skillet sprayed with nonstick spray. Turn the pancakes when bubbles appear on the surface; cook for 1 more minute.

For one serving, spread 3 pancakes with all fruit jam or fruit syrup. Top with mixed berries. Freeze any leftovers in individual freezer bags. When ready to use, toast the pancakes to thaw and heat. Each serving gives 1½ complex carbohydrate (oats), 2 ounces protein (ricotta and eggwhites), and 1 simple carbohydrate (fruit and fruit jam)

Makes 12 3-inch pancakes

Per serving: 35 grams carbohydrate; 12 grams protein; 7 grams fat; 26 percent calories from fat, 3 milligrams cholesterol, 97.5 milligrams sodium, 251 calories.

SOUTHWESTERN FRUIT TOAST

2 egg whites, lightly beaten
2 tablespoons skim milk
1 teaspoons vanilla
1 10-inch whole wheat flour tortilla
nonstick cooking spray
2 tablespoons Grape-Nuts or low-fat granola
½ cup mixed berries
1 tablespoon all-fruit pourable syrup

Beat together the egg whites, milk, and vanilla. Dip the tortilla into the mixture, letting it absorb the liquid for a minute or so. Coat a nonstick skillet with nonstick spray and heat. Gently lift the tortilla with a spatula, place it in the skillet and cook until it is golden brown on each side. Sprinkle one half of the tortilla with cereal and berries. Fold the tortilla over omelette style and slide it onto a plate. Drizzle it with all-fruit syrup. Gives 2 complex carbohydrates (tortilla and cereal), 2 ounces protein (milk and egg whites), and 1 simple carbohydrate (fruit and fruit syrup)

Serves 1

Per serving: 44 grams carbohydrate; 13.5 grams protein; 2 grams fat; 7 percent calories from fat, 8 milligrams cholesterol, 266 milligrams sodium, 249 calories.

ORANGE VANILLA FRENCH TOAST

4 egg whites, lightly beaten
½ teaspoon ground cinnamon
½ cup skim milk
4 slices whole wheat bread
2 tablespoons frozen, unsweetened orange juice concentrate, undiluted
4 tablespoons all-fruit jam or pourable syrup
1 teaspoons vanilla
nonstick cooking spray

Beat together the egg whites, milk, orange juice concentrate, vanilla, and cinnamon. Add the bread slices one at a time, letting the bread absorb the liquid; this may take a few minutes. Coat a skillet with nonstick cooking spray and heat. Gently lift each bread slice with a spatula and place it in the skillet; cook on each side until golden brown. Serve each slice of toast topped with 1 tablespoon all-fruit jam or all-fruit pourable syrup. Freeze the leftovers in individual freezer bags. When ready to use a slice, toast it to thaw and heat. Each serving gives 1 complex carbohydrate (bread), 1 ounce protein (egg whites and milk), and 1 simple carbohydrate (juice and all-fruit jam).

Serves 4

Per serving: 28 grams carbohydrate; 8 grams protein; 1.5 grams fat; 11 percent calories from fat; 2 milligrams cholesterol; 250 milligrams sodium; 152 calories

BAKED BREAKFAST APPLE

1 small Golden Delicious apple, cored

1 tablespoon raisins

2 tablespoons old-fashioned oats

2 tablespoons apple juice

$\frac{1}{4}$ teaspoon cinnamon

$\frac{1}{2}$ cup nonfat ricotta cheese

Place the apple in a microwavable bowl. Mix together oats, cinnamon, and raisins. Fill the cavity of the cored apple with the mixture. Pour the apple juice over the apple, and cover it with plastic wrap. Microwave on high for 1 minute. Turn the dish around halfway and microwave for 1 minute more. Spoon the ricotta cheese onto a plate, and top it with the apple and the heated juice mixture. Gives 1 complex carbohydrate (oats), 2 ounces protein (ricotta), and 1 simple carbohydrate (apple, juice, and raisins).

Serves 1

Per serving: 30 grams carbohydrate; 14 grams protein; 1 grams fat; 6 percent calories from fat; 23 milligrams cholesterol; 100 milligrams sodium; 183 calories

BREAKFAST SUNDAE SUPREME

$\frac{1}{2}$ banana, quartered lengthwise

$\frac{1}{4}$ cup crushed unsweetened pineapple

$\frac{1}{2}$ cup nonfat ricotta cheese

2 tablespoons Grape-Nuts or low-fat granola

$\frac{1}{4}$ cup strawberries, sliced

1 teaspoon honey or all-fruit pourable syrup

Place the banana quarters star-fashion on a small plate. Scoop ricotta cheese onto the center points. Surround with the other fruit; then sprinkle with cereal. Drizzle with honey or all-fruit syrup. Gives 1 complex carbohydrate (cereal), 2 ounces protein (ricotta), and 2 simple carbohydrates (fruit).

Serves 1

Per serving: 42 grams carbohydrate; 15 grams protein; 1 gram fat; 4 percent calories from fat; 5 milligrams cholesterol; 111 milligrams sodium; 224 calories

HOT APPLE CINNAMON OATMEAL

$^2/_3$ cup old-fashioned oats

1 teaspoon vanilla

1$^1/_2$ cups skim milk

$^1/_2$ teaspoon cinnamon

$^1/_2$ cup apple or white grape juice, unsweetened

$^1/_2$ teaspoon pumpkin pie spice

2 tablespoons raisins, dark or golden

In a small pot, bring the oats, milk, and juice to a boil. Cook for 5 minutes, stirring occasionally. Add raisins, vanilla, cinnamon, and pumpkin pie spice. Remove from heat, cover the pot and let the oats sit for 2 to 3 minutes to thicken. Combine all ingredients and cook for 5 to 6 minutes on high. Gives 1 complex carbohydrate (oats), 1 ounce protein (milk), and 1 simple carbohydrate (juice and raisins).

Serves 2

Per Serving: 29 grams carbohydrate; 11 grams protein; 1 gram fat; 5 percent calories from fat; 3 milligrams cholesterol; 97 milligrams sodium; 169 calories

My Quickest Lunches

1. Cheese Quesadillas: Fat-free whole-wheat tortilla sprinkled with two ounces of shredded part-skim cheddar cheese and drizzled with salsa, then folded and browned in a nonstick skillet until cheese melts. Serve with apple slices.

2. Baked Spaghetti: Cooked whole-wheat angel hair pasta in a sheet pan, topped with one jar of Classico Tomato Basil Sauce, sprinkled with one pound of shredded mozzarella cheese, and baked for eight to ten minutes on 375 degrees. One 3 x 5 portion (index card size) is approximately one serving. Serve with "salad in a bag" with low-fat vinaigrette.

3. **Vegetable Tortilla Pizza:** Large whole wheat flour tortilla brushed with Classico Tomato Basil Sauce, topped with chopped veggies of choice, and sprinkled with grated mozzarella. Bake until lightly browned and crisp (about 5 minutes) at 450 degrees. Serve with baby carrots to munch on.

4. **Grilled Chicken Sandwich:** Grilled marinated chicken breast (from your freezer) on whole-grain bun with lettuce, tomato, salsa, or Dijon mustard. Serve with fresh fruit.

5. **Turkey and White Bean Soup:** Smoked turkey breast (pre-cooked) made into soup with chicken stock and cannelini beans. Serve with raw veggies and fruit.

6. **Quick Taco Salad:** Canned black beans, rinsed, then spiced with creole seasoning and sprinkled with shredded part-skim cheddar cheese. Heat and serve over mixed greens and crumbled baked Tostitos with salsa. Serve with sliced oranges.

7. **Even Quicker Greek Salad:** Mixed greens (from a bag), topped with crumbled feta cheese and shredded Boar's Head turkey or ham, and drizzled with low-fat vinaigrette. Serve with toasted petite whole wheat pita and a piece of fruit.

8. **Cheese-Baked Potatoes:** Microwave potatoes for four minutes each, then cut open and top with cooked broccoli florets and Laughing Cow Lite Wedges (two per potato) or two ounces of another part-skim cheese. Microwave again until cheese melts. Top with nonfat sour cream or salsa. Serve with salad and low-fat vinaigrette.

SMART WEIGH EATING TIPS

- **Plan ahead.** An empty fridge after a stressful day begs for pizza. Don't leave meals to chance.
- **Stock frozen veggies.** With pasta or stir-fry sauces, they are quick and healthy meals.
- **Don't give in to peer pressure.** If the cookies, chips, or ice cream you buy for the rest of the family is sabotaging your efforts, stop buying them.
- **Enlist professional help.** Registered dietitians, certified personal trainers, and psychologists can help you deal with problems hindering your efforts. If you feel like you can't do it on your own, seek help.

Deliciously Simple Dinners

Pasta Shrimp Pomodoro with Fresh Broccoli Salad
shrimp (protein) • pasta (complex carbohydrate) • broccoli (simple carbohydrate)

PASTA SHRIMP POMODORO

1 ½ pounds shrimp, peeled and deveined

¼ cup white wine Worcestershire sauce

8 ounces dry angel hair pasta

2 teaspoons olive oil

2 cloves garlic, minced

1 small red onion, chopped

1 each yellow, orange, and red bell peppers, cut into strips

1 teaspoon Mrs. Dash seasoning

1 teaspoon creole seasoning

1 teaspoon dried oregano

½ teaspoon dried basil

1 can (32 ounces) whole tomatoes

2 tablespoons grated Parmesan cheese

Marinate shrimp in Worcestershire sauce for at least 15 minutes.

In a large saucepan, cook pasta in salted water until done. Drain.

Spray a nonstick skillet with cooking spray. Lightly sauté half of the garlic and half of the onions. Add shrimp and sear on one side for 1 minute; then turn and sear on other side.

Spray another skillet with cooking spray and add olive oil; heat. Add remaining garlic and onions, sauté. Then add peppers, seasonings and herbs. Allow peppers to soften, then add tomatoes, breaking up tomatoes with spatula while heating. Allow to simmer and reduce for about 4 to 5 minutes. Add shrimp, stirring all together. Sprinkle with Parmesan cheese. Serve over cooked pasta.

Serves 4

FRESH BROCCOLI SALAD

2 bunches fresh broccoli, trimmed and cut into small pieces

1 cup chopped fresh parsley

2 to 3 green onions, sliced

½ cup nonfat cottage cheese (or ricotta)

¼ cup light mayonnaise

½ cup skim milk

2 cloves garlic, minced

1 teaspoon Mrs. Dash seasoning

½ teaspoon creole seasoning

¾ teaspoon dill weed

Blanch broccoli for 5 minutes in boiling water. Immerse quickly in ice water to chill; drain. Toss with parsley and green onions.

Make dressing by blending cottage cheese, mayonnaise, milk, garlic, and seasonings in blender until smooth. Stir in dill. Toss with vegetables and chill well.
Serves 8

Herb-Crusted Orange Roughy with Herb-Roasted Potatoes

fish (protein) • potatoes, bread crumbs (complex carbohydrate) • broccoli (simple carbohydrate)

HERB-CRUSTED ORANGE ROUGHY

4 orange roughy fillets (5 ounces each)

¼ cup white wine Worcestershire sauce

1 teaspoon creole seasoning

½ cup dried bread crumbs (purchased)

2 tablespoons chopped fresh herbs (cilantro, basil, rosemary, thyme)

¼ cup Dijon mustard

2 cups broccoli florets, steamed until crisp tender

½ cup Tomato Basil Sauce (recipe follows)

1 tablespoon parsley, chopped

Marinate orange roughy in Worcestershire sauce for at least 15 minutes, or up to 1 hour.

Preheat oven to 375 degrees.

Season fish with seasoning and roll in bread crumbs. Spread mustard on top of fish and roll in bread crumbs once more.

Spray a nonstick skillet with cooking spray; heat. Sear fish in hot skillet on both sides, then transfer to oven and roast until done and browned.

Serve on bed of tomato basil sauce with steamed broccoli. Sprinkle with chopped parsley.
Serves 4

TOMATO BASIL SAUCE

1 tablespoon olive oil

2 white onions, diced medium

2 teaspoons minced garlic

½ cup minced shallots

1 tablespoon chopped fresh thyme

1 teaspoon chopped fresh rosemary

1 tablespoon chopped fresh oregano

2 tablespoons chopped fresh basil

5 tomatoes, skinned, seeded, and diced*

1 can (32 ounces) whole tomatoes

1 tablespoon creole seasoning

1 tablespoon Mrs. Dash Garlic and Herb seasoning

Sauté onions, garlic, shallots, and herbs in olive oil until onions are transparent, about 3 to 4 minutes. Add fresh and canned tomatoes. Cook for 5 minutes at full heat. Lower heat and continue cooking until sauce has reduced by one-third.

Add seasonings. Cook for about 1½ hours, stirring occasionally. Leave chunky; do not grind or blend.

This sauce may be made in large quantities and frozen (after cooling) in zip-top bags for later use. Microwave or place in refrigerator to thaw.

*Tomatoes are easily skinned by immersing them in boiling water for 10 seconds. Remove with slotted spoon. Skins will "slip off."

Makes 14 ½-cup servings

HERB-ROASTED POTATOES

2 pounds (about 5 large) red-skinned potatoes, scrubbed and quartered

2 cloves garlic, minced

2 teaspoons olive oil

½ teaspoon creole seasoning

1 teaspoon Mrs. Dash seasoning

1 tablespoon chopped fresh rosemary (or 1 teaspoon dried)

Preheat oven to 450 degrees.

Spray a shallow roasting pan with cooking spray. Add potatoes, garlic, olive oil, seasonings, and rosemary, and spread in an even layer. Bake until the potatoes begin to brown, 20 to 30 minutes, turning them once midway through roasting.

Serves 4

Seared Pork Tenderloin with Cinnamon Sweet Potatoes and Fresh Asparagus

pork (protein) • sweet potatoes (complex carbohydrate) • asparagus (simple carbohydrate)

SEARED PORK TENDERLOIN

1½ pounds pork tenderloin, trimmed of all visible fat

½ cup white wine Worcestershire sauce

½ teaspoon creole seasoning

2 tablespoon chopped fresh herbs (cilantro, basil, rosemary, thyme)

1 teaspoon Mrs. Dash seasoning

2 garlic cloves, minced

1 large red onion, sliced thin

Preheat oven to 400 degrees.

Marinate pork tenderloin in Worcester-shire sauce, seasonings, herbs, and garlic for at least 1 hour.

Sear pork on both sides in hot ovenproof skillet, then top with sliced onions. Place whole skillet in oven for 15 minutes or until internal temperature reaches 150 to 170 degrees. May pour on additional marinade while roasting.

Serves 4

CINNAMON SWEET POTATOES

4 sweet potatoes

cinnamon

Preheat oven to 400 degrees.

Wash and scrub sweet potatoes. Place in oven for 35 minutes. (You may add the skillet of pork tenderloins to the oven after 20 minutes.)

Cut open sweet potatoes and push ends together to "mash" toward center and fluff. Sprinkle with cinnamon.

Serves 4

FRESH ASPARAGUS

1 pound fresh asparagus, trimmed

¼ cup chicken stock (fat-free/low salt)

1 teaspoon Mrs. Dash seasoning

½ teaspoon creole seasoning

Microwave asparagus in chicken stock and seasonings for about 7 to 8 minutes or until crisp tender.

Serves 4

Chicken Laurent with Brown Rice Pilaf

chicken (protein) • rice (complex carbohydrate) • asparagus, red onion (simple carbohydrate)

CHICKEN LAURENT

4 boneless, skinless chicken breast halves (1 pound)
$\frac{1}{4}$ cup white wine Worcestershire sauce
2 teaspoons olive oil
2 cloves garlic, minced
2 teaspoons shallots, minced
1 teaspoon Mrs. Dash seasoning
$\frac{1}{2}$ teaspoon creole seasoning
1 pound asparagus, trimmed
1 red onion, sliced thin
$\frac{1}{3}$ cup white wine*
$\frac{2}{3}$ cup chicken stock (fat-free/low salt)
2 teaspoons cornstarch
*or substitute dealcoholized wine or more chicken stock

Preheat oven to 375 degrees.

Marinate chicken breasts in Worcester-shire sauce for at least 15 minutes.

Place asparagus spears with $\frac{1}{4}$ cup water in a glass baking dish; cover with vented plastic wrap. Microwave on high to blanch for 3 to 4 minutes.

Spray nonstick ovenproof skillet with cooking spray. Add olive oil and heat. Add garlic and shallots to pan; lightly sauté. Add marinated chicken breasts and brown on both sides, sprinkling with seasonings. Lay asparagus and red onion slices on top of chicken.

Stir together wine and chicken stock in a small stock pot; add cornstarch mixed with 1 tablespoon cold water. Stir over moderate heat until thickened. Pour over chicken and vegetables.

Bake in oven for 30 minutes.

Serves 4

BROWN RICE PILAF

1 teaspoon olive oil
$\frac{1}{2}$ red onion, diced
2 cloves garlic, minced
$1\frac{3}{4}$ cups chicken stock (fat-free/low salt)
$\frac{1}{2}$ teaspoon creole seasoning
1 tablespoon chopped fresh herbs (cilantro, basil, rosemary, thyme)
2 cups instant brown rice

Spray a medium saucepan with cooking spray; add olive oil and heat. Add diced onion and garlic, and lightly sauté about 1 to 2 minutes; then add chicken stock, seasoning and herbs.

Let mixture come to a boil, then stir in brown rice. Let boil for 1 minute, turn down heat to low and cover. Let simmer for 5 minutes, uncover skillet, and fluff rice with fork. Cover again. Let sit for another 5 minutes.
Serves 6

Chicken Paella with Spicy Tomato and Cucumber Salad

chicken (protein) • rice, peas (complex carbohydrate) • tomato, cucumbers (simple carbohydrate)

CHICKEN PAELLA

1 pound boneless, skinless chicken breast, trimmed of fat and cut into chunks
$\frac{1}{4}$ cup white wine Worcestershire sauce
2 teaspoons olive oil
2 cloves garlic, minced
1 small onion, diced
1 cup arborio (or medium grain) rice
2 cups chicken stock (fat-free/low salt)
$\frac{1}{4}$ teaspoon crushed saffron threads (or $\frac{1}{8}$ teaspoon powdered)
$\frac{1}{2}$ teaspoon creole seasoning
1 teaspoon Mrs. Dash seasoning
1 cup frozen peas, thawed
$\frac{1}{3}$ cup jarred, roasted red peppers, drained and cut into strips

Marinate chicken breasts in Worcestershire sauce for up to 1 hour.
Spray a large nonstick skillet with cooking spray. Add olive oil and heat over

medium-high heat. Add garlic and onions and sauté 30 seconds, then add marinated chicken chunks. Sauté until slightly browned on the outside and opaque inside, 3 to 4 minutes. Remove chicken from skillet and set aside.

To skillet, add rice and stir to coat well. Stir in chicken stock, saffron, and seasonings. Cover and cook over low heat for 20 minutes. Gently stir in cooked chicken, green peas, and roasted red peppers. Cover again and cook, stirring occasionally, until rice is tender, about 5 minutes more. Serve immediately.
Serves 4

SPICY TOMATO AND CUCUMBER SALAD

> 2 large tomatoes, cut into wedges
> 1 cup diced cucumber
> $\frac{1}{2}$ cup finely chopped red onion
> 1 clove garlic, minced
> 2 tablespoons chopped fresh cilantro
> 2 tablespoons red wine vinegar
> 2 teaspoons chopped fresh hot green chili pepper
>   (or $\frac{1}{4}$ teaspoon crushed red pepper)
> 1 teaspoon honey
> $\frac{1}{2}$ teaspoon creole seasoning

In a medium-sized bowl, mix together all ingredients. Cover and refrigerate about 2 hours or until chilled.
Serves 6

Poached Salmon Over Black Beans and Corn with Apple Walnut Salad

*salmon, black beans (protein) • corn, black beans (complex carbohydrate) •
vegetables, fruit (simple carbohydrate)*

POACHED SALMON
> 4 salmon fillets (4 ounces each)
POACHING STOCK
> 1 cup white wine*
> 2 cups chicken stock (fat free/low salt)
> 1 whole shallot, quartered
> 2 cloves garlic, minced
> 2 sprigs fresh thyme

2 bay leaves

¼ teaspoon cracked black pepper

½ teaspoon creole seasoning

1 pound asparagus, trimmed of tough stalks

2 cups Black Bean and Corn Salsa (recipe follows)

2 cups fresh spinach leaves, washed and stemmed

1 tablespoon chopped chives

1 lemon, sliced

*or substitute nonalcoholic wine or more chicken stock

In a large nonstick skillet, bring poaching stock to boil. Add salmon and asparagus spears; simmer 5 to 7 minutes until done.

Spoon Black Bean and Corn Salsa onto plate. Add fresh spinach leaves and place poached salmon and asparagus spears on top of the leaves.

Sprinkle with chopped chives and garnish with twisted lemon slice.

Serves 4

BLACK BEAN AND CORN SALSA

2 cups black beans, drained and rinsed

1 cup frozen corn kernels, thawed

2 plum tomatoes, diced

½ red onion, minced

1 serrano pepper, minced

1 tablespoon chopped fresh cilantro

1 tablespoon olive oil

4 cloves garlic, minced

juice of 2 limes

1 tablespoon balsamic vinegar

1 teaspoon cumin

2 teaspoons hot pepper sauce

1 teaspoon creole seasoning

In a large bowl, combine all ingredients and mix well. Allow to marinate at least one hour before serving.

Makes 10 ⅓-cup servings

APPLE WALNUT SALAD

2 Granny Smith apples, cored and sliced thin

2 tablespoons chopped walnuts

2 tablespoons chicken stock
(fat free/low salt)
1 tablespoon white wine vinegar
2 teaspoons walnut oil (or olive oil)
1 tablespoon finely chopped shallots
1 teaspoon Dijon mustard
$\frac{1}{4}$ teaspoon salt
$\frac{1}{4}$ teaspoon cracked black pepper
8 cups washed, dried, and torn mixed greens
   (red leaf, romaine, frisee, radicchio, arugula, or bibb)

In a small, dry skillet over low heat, stir walnuts until lightly toasted, about 3 minutes. Transfer to a plate to cool.

In a large salad bowl, whisk together chicken stock, vinegar, oil, shallots, mustard, salt, and pepper. Add greens and apples and toss thoroughly. Sprinkle with the toasted walnuts.

Serves 4

Red Lentil Chili with Southwest Cornbread and Crunchy Jicama and Melon Salad

lentils, cheese (protein) • lentils, cornbread (complex carbohydrate) • vegetables, salad (simple carbohydrate)

RED LENTIL CHILI

$\frac{1}{2}$ pound carrots
1 small zucchini
1 small yellow squash
$\frac{1}{2}$ large eggplant
$\frac{1}{2}$ large red onion
$\frac{3}{4}$ tablespoon olive oil
12-ounce bag red or brown lentils, rinsed
2 cups chicken stock (fat free/low salt)
1 teaspoon Mrs. Dash seasoning
1 teaspoon creole seasoning
2 bay leaves
$\frac{1}{2}$ tablespoon oregano
$\frac{1}{2}$ teaspoon cumin
1 teaspoon chili powder
$\frac{3}{4}$ teaspoon cayenne

$\frac{3}{4}$ teaspoon nutmeg

2 cloves garlic, minced

1 jalapeño pepper, chopped

2 cans (32 ounces each) plum tomatoes

In food processor, finely chop carrots, zucchini, squash, eggplant, and onion. Spray nonstick skillet with cooking spray. Add olive oil. Heat over medium high heat. Add chopped vegetables. Sauté for 5 minutes. Add lentils, chicken stock, seasonings, herbs, spices, garlic, jalapeño peppers and tomatoes. Simmer for 2 hours.
Serves 10 (1½ cups each)

SOUTHWEST CORNBREAD

2 tablespoons canola oil

$\frac{1}{2}$ cup finely chopped onion

1 egg, lightly beaten

1 tablespoon honey

1 cup skim milk

1 cup whole wheat pastry flour

1 cup yellow cornmeal

1 tablespoon baking powder

1$\frac{1}{2}$ teaspoon salt

1 cup fresh or frozen corn

$\frac{1}{2}$ cup shredded part-skim cheddar cheese

Preheat oven to 375 degrees.

Heat oil in a small skillet. Add onion and sauté for 5 to 8 minutes or until onion is soft.

Beat together egg, honey, and milk; set aside.

In a separate bowl, combine flour, cornmeal, baking powder, and salt. Add to liquid mixture. Add corn, shredded cheese and onions along with all excess oil. Mix well. Spread into an 8-inch square pan coated with cooking spray.

Bake for 25 to 35 minutes or until brown and firm on top. Cut into 16 pieces.
Serves 16

CRUNCHY JICAMA AND MELON SALAD

1 medium jicama, julienned

1 medium cantaloupe, cut into $\frac{1}{2}$ inch cubes

3 tablespoons lime juice

3 tablespoons chopped fresh mint (or 1 tablespoon dried)

1 teaspoon grated lime peel

2 teaspoons honey

$\frac{1}{4}$ teaspoon salt

In a medium-sized bowl, mix together all ingredients. Cover and refrigerate 2 hours or until chilled.

Serves 4

Risotto with Spring Vegetables and Mixed Greens with Citrus Vinaigrette

cheeses (protein) • rice (complex carbohydrate) • salad (simple carbohydrate)

RISOTTO WITH SPRING VEGETABLES

$5\frac{1}{2}$ to $6\frac{1}{2}$ cups chicken stock (fat free/low salt)

16 baby carrots, shaved and cut in half

8 medium stalks asparagus, trimmed and cut into 2-inch pieces

1 cup sugar snap peas (thawed if frozen)

1 red bell pepper, cut into strips

2 teaspoons olive oil

2 cloves garlic, minced

1 red onion, diced

1 cup arborio or medium grain

rice, uncooked

$\frac{1}{2}$ cup white wine*

$\frac{1}{2}$ teaspoon creole seasoning

$1\frac{1}{2}$ tablespoons chopped fresh basil

$\frac{1}{2}$ cup grated Parmesan cheese

2 tablespoons chopped fresh herbs (cilantro, basil, rosemary, thyme)

*or substitute dealcoholized wine or more chicken stock

In a medium-sized stockpot, bring chicken stock to boil over medium heat. Add carrots and cook 3 to 5 minutes until almost tender. Add asparagus and snap peas, and cook 1 minute longer. Remove vegetables with slotted spoon and place in bowl to cool. Reduce heat and keep stock simmering.

Spray a nonstick skillet with cooking spray. Add olive oil; heat. Add garlic and onions, and sauté until translucent, about 3 minutes. Add rice and stir to coat grains. Add wine and cook until most of liquid has been absorbed, about 2 to 3 minutes. Add $\frac{1}{2}$ cup simmering chicken stock and cook another 2 to 3 minutes.

Continue adding stock, ½ cup at a time, until rice begins to soften, about 15 minutes.

Stir in the seasoning and basil, adding more stock to keep mixture creamy. Stir in reserved vegetables and cheese. Sprinkle with herbs.

Serves 4

MIXED GREENS WITH CITRUS VINAIGRETTE

12 cups washed, dried, and torn mixed greens
   (red leaf, romaine, frisee, radicchio, arugula, or bibb)
½ cup Citrus Vinaigrette (recipe follows)
4 green onions, leaves curled
2 tablespoons chopped fresh herbs (cilantro, basil, rosemary, thyme)
2 plum tomatoes, diced

Just before serving, toss lettuce leaves with Citrus Vinaigrette. Top with curly-leaved onion and sprinkle lightly with herbs and diced tomatoes.

Serves 4

CITRUS VINAIGRETTE

2 tablespoons olive oil
⅔ cup rice wine vinegar
⅓ cup orange juice
1 tablespoon Dijon mustard
1 teaspoon honey
2 teaspoons minced garlic
1 tablespoon minced shallots
½ teaspoon creole seasoning
2 tablespoons chopped fresh cilantro

Mix all ingredients together. Refrigerate.

Serves 12

CHAPTER 11

SMART WEIGH
DINING OUT
AND TRAVEL GUIDE

IF IT SEEMS AS IF YOU HARDLY eat at home anymore, you're not alone. The home-cooked meal is not yet an endangered species, but meals prepared and eaten at home are at an all-time low. One nationwide analysis of American eating habits found that almost half of all U.S. food dollars are spent eating away from home.

In the last decade of the twentieth century alone, dining in restaurants increased by 14 percent—and fast food restaurants captured more than 80 percent of that growth in the past five years. Every day 160 million people eat out at restaurants and 2 million children eat at one of the three major burger joints. Each day, 100 million M&Ms are downed, along with 30 million hot dogs. No wonder we're in the shape we're in!

But I can't always eat at home, you might be thinking. No, most of us in the twenty-first century are on the run, and having every meal at our own dining room table is unrealistic. But the typical scenario when dining out is to eat too much of the wrong foods prepared in unhealthy ways. In a small study of 129 women, researchers at the University of Memphis and Vanderbilt University found that those who ate out more than five times a week consumed an average of 2,056 calories per day, compared with an average of 1,768 calories for those who ate out five or fewer times a week. That may not sound like much, but that higher calorie consumption could add up to two to three pounds on your body *every month*—or as much as 24 to 36 additional pounds a year!

The challenge as you choose to dine out The Smart Weigh is to enjoy fine food without compromising health and weight. The main threats to healthy dining lie mostly in the "hidden fats" of restaurant preparation. A typical restaurant meal packs in the equivalent of twelve to fourteen pats of butter. To sidestep some of the land mines of eating out, follow these guidelines.

Dining Out The Smart Weigh

Plan Ahead

Choose a restaurant that you know and trust for quality food and a willingness to prepare foods in a healthful way upon request. Many progressive and responsible restaurants have begun to offer healthy menu selections—recognizing that healthy eating is not a passing fad.

Order Smart

Never be timid about ordering foods prepared according to your needs. After all, you are paying (and paying well) for the meal and service. You also have a right to know the content of what you are going to eat. Remember, it's your health, your money, and your waistline—so speak up! Don't be intimidated by the waiters or chef; they generally want to please you.

Most foods can be prepared without fat and butter; just order meats, poultry, or fish grilled without butter or oils, and request sauces on the side. Good choices: marinated, grilled breast of chicken, grilled or broiled fish or seafood, and steamed shellfish. Entrées that are poached in wine or lemon juice are good options as well as those simmered in tomato sauces.

When fresh vegetables are available, order them steamed without added butter or sauces. When ordering salad dressing for salads, mayonnaise for sandwiches, butter or sour cream for a potato, ask for it on the side, and apply it in limited quantities. For example, lightly drizzle 1 tablespoon of dressing on your salad for flavor, and use extra vinegar or lemon juice for moisture.

Watch Your Portions

The typical restaurant serves twice as much as you need. And believe me, as an adult there are no rewards for cleaning your plate. You can make better choices: ordering appetizers instead of entrées, lunch portions at dinner, sharing a meal with a willing partner, or taking home leftovers for a great meal tomorrow.

When making your meal choices, don't give meat the starring role. A healthy serving of meat is the size of a computer mouse or a deck

---

FAT-LADEN WORDS

Restaurant menus give you plenty of clues about what the selections contain. Avoid items with these words attached.

If you see these words, be bold enough to ask for the entrée prepared in a healthful way; that is, if the description says "buttered," ask for it without added butter; if the description says "pan-fried," ask for it grilled or poached instead.

- à la mode *(with ice cream)*
- au fromage *(with cheese)*
- au gratin *(in cheese sauce)*
- au lait *(with milk)*
- basted *(with extra fat)*
- bisque *(cream soup)*
- buttered *(with extra fat)*
- casserole *(with extra fat)*
- creamed *(with extra fat)*
- crispy *(means fried)*
- escalloped *(with cream sauce)*
- pan-fried *(fried with extra fat)*
- hash *(with extra fat)*
- hollandaise *(with cream sauce)*
- sautéed *(fried with extra fat)*

of cards. You'll get the right foods in the right proportions for a healthy meal every time if half of your plate holds veggies, one quarter holds the protein serving, and the other quarter holds the starchy foods (rice, pasta, or potatoes).

Have a carbohydrate and a protein at each meal, never just a salad. You may order a chef's salad with extra turkey rather than ham, or a shrimp cocktail with your salad; but be sure to include a protein. Many salad bars offer protein sources in cottage cheese, grated cheese, or chopped eggs. Your carbohydrate may be a roll, crackers, or baked potato.

Finally, guard against the desire to eat all you can at all-you-can-eat brunches, buffets, or even salad bars. Your overeating ("I want to get my money's worth") is not going to cheat the restaurant out of anything, but it can cheat you out of many healthy years.

Eat-Smart Ideas

Let's look at the good and bad qualities of various cuisines and restaurants. Use this guide to help you make better choices when eating away from home.

MEXICAN

Ask that a salad be served immediately (with dressing on the side) in place of the chips. It will help prevent the "munch a bunch" syndrome. And don't eat the fried tortilla shell your salad may be served in; those shells are grease sponges with upwards of twenty-two grams of fat per shell.

Always order à la carte rather than a combo plate, which is often laden with high-fat side dishes such as refried beans (refried beans are made with pure lard). You can also request that the sour cream and cheese toppings be omitted from your dish. These carry ten grams of fat per ounce.

And beware of the margaritas—they are loaded with both salt and sugar, to say nothing of alcohol!

Smart choices: black bean soup; chili or gazpacho; chicken burrito, tostada, or enchilada; soft chicken tacos; chicken fajitas (without added fat).

ASIAN

Chinese, Korean, Thai, or Vietnamese food are excellent choices for dining out because stir-frying is the main method of cooking. This terrific technique cooks the vegetables quickly, retaining the nutrients, and, if requested, uses very little oil.

Order dishes that have been lightly stir-fried (not deep-fried like egg rolls) and are without heavy gravies or sweet-and-sour sauces. Half a dinner portion is appropriate, with steamed brown or white rice; fried rice is just that—fried!

Many restaurants will prepare food without MSG if you ask, and be careful to watch the soy sauce you add. Both are loaded with sodium.

Sushi is awesome for the enthusiast, but be sure you are eating it at a high-quality restaurant that is serving the freshest fish from the best sources. If in doubt, have grilled teriyaki instead.

Smart choices: bamboo-steamed vegetables with chicken, seafood, or fish; Moo Goo Gai Pan; shrimp or tofu with vegetables (with no MSG and little oil); wonton, hot and sour, or miso soup; udon noodles with meat and vegetables; Yakitori (meats broiled on skewers).

ITALIAN

Controlling the size of the portion is especially important here; the typical plate of spaghetti is five times too much. Although pasta with red sauce is a relatively low-fat choice, order it in a side dish or appetizer portion topped with steamed or grilled seafood, chicken, or fish. Ask for your salad with dressing on the side, and never hesitate to request a red sauce rather than a butter or white sauce.

Smart choices: grilled chicken with a pasta side dish or bread; fresh fish with pasta side dish or bread; clam linguine with red sauce (be careful about the amount of pasta); grilled shrimp on fettucine with red sauce; Cioppino (seafood soup); minestrone soup and salad (dressing on side), with à la carte mozzarella cheese or meatballs for protein; side dish of spaghetti with two à la carte meatballs.

SEAFOOD

When possible, order fresh fish or seafood steamed, boiled, grilled, or broiled without butter. A small amount of cocktail sauce is a better choice for dipping than butter (two dips in butter = fifty calories). Remember that small seafood items such as shrimp, oysters, etc., are deadly in terms of fat and calories when fried; the surface area is so high that more breading adheres and absorbs more fat.

Smart choices: fresh fish of the day—grilled when possible, without butter, sauce on the side; steamed oysters, shrimp, or clams; lobster/crabmeat/crab claws; seafood kabobs; mesquite grilled shrimp; blackened fish or seafood from the grill, prepared without butter.

STEAK HOUSES

Portion control is also crucial here. A sixteen-ounce steak or prime rib will give you far more protein and fat than you need. Order the smallest cut available, and plan on taking some home.

Smart choices: petite cut filet; shish-ka-bob or brochette; slices of London broil (no sauces); Hawaiian chicken or marinated grilled chicken breast; charbroiled shrimp (grilled without butter).

HEALTH/NATURAL FOOD RESTAURANTS

Do not feel "safe" here by any means! Although you will have an opportunity to get whole grains and nicer fresh vegetable salads, you still need to avoid the fats and sodium. Many foods are prepared in the same way at "health food" restaurants as at the drive-through; they just have healthier sounding names. Beware of sauces and high-fat cheeses smothering the foods, as well as high-fat dressings on salads and sandwiches. If you have a cheese dish, be sure to use no other added fats in the meal; the cheese will contain enough for the day.

Smart choices: vegetable soup and ½ sandwich (avoid tuna/chicken salad due to mayo); "chef"-type salad (no ham) and whole grain roll; stir-fry dishes, asking for "light" on oil; marinated breast of chicken; fresh fish of the day, grilled when possible; vegetable omelet with whole-grain roll; pita stuffed with vegetables and cheese; fruit plate with plain yogurt/cottage cheese and whole-grain roll.

FAST FOOD RESTAURANTS

If you have to eat in a hurry and can't request special preparation for a sit-down meal, at least become more aware of the hidden fats in the foods you consider while you're on the run.

- Special sauces: it's the mayonnaise, special sauces, sour cream, etc., that triple the fat, sodium, and calories in fast foods. Always order your take-out without them.
- Stuffed potatoes may seem a healthy addition to the fast food menu, but not if they're smothered in cheese sauce (equivalent to nine pats of butter per potato). Ask for grated cheese, and no butter, instead.
- Chicken is a lower-fat alternative than beef, but not when it's batter-fried. One serving of chicken nuggets has the equivalent of five pats of butter—more than twice what you would get in a regular hamburger. And the fat it's soaked in is purely saturated—usually just melted beef fat. A chicken sandwich is no health package either—it usually has enough fat to equal eleven pats of butter, unless the chicken is grilled.
- Croissant sandwiches aren't a whole lot more than a meal on a grease bun. Most take-out croissants have the equivalent of more than four pats of butter, and the toppings add insult to injury.
- Salad bars can add fiber and nutrients to a meal, but it's only salad vegetables that do so. The mayonnaise-based salads, croutons, and bacon bits should be left on the bar, and dressing used sparingly. Use extra lemon juice or vinegar instead.
- Frozen yogurt, although lower in fat and cholesterol than ice

cream, contains more sugar, so it is not a perfectly healthy substitute. This also applies to frozen tofu desserts. Substitute one
of the new sorbet-like frozen desserts that are primarily fruit.
They will contain some sugar, but usually not in such high
amounts.

While many unhealthy foods await you in the fast food lane,
some are also available that can make eating "fast" a part of your
Smart Weigh plan. Use this guide to help you eat smarter at the
take-out counter.

Burger King: Although no burger is truly lean, the smaller the portion, the less fat you get. A Whopper Jr. without mayonnaise is filling and tasty and delivers twenty-five fewer grams of fat than the
regular Whopper. Also try the B.K. Broiler Chicken Sandwich (without dressing or mayonnaise; try barbecue sauce for a bit of extra flavor) or Chunky Chicken Salad with reduced-calorie Italian dressing
and your own whole-grain crackers or whole-grain bread.

Wendy's: Order a plain baked potato (without cheese sauce—get
a side of chili instead as a topping). Or try the salad bar, filling up
on raw vegetables rather than potato or macaroni salad, etc; use garbanzo beans or chili for protein. Other smart choices include the Jr.
Hamburger (without mayonnaise), Grilled Chicken or Spicy Chicken
Filet Sandwich, Chicken Caesar Pita (without the dressing), Garden
Veggie Pita (without the dressing), or Caesar Side Salad (without the
dressing) topped with Grilled Chicken using reduced-fat and low-
calorie Italian dressing instead of the Caesar.

McDonald's: Choose the Grilled Chicken Deluxe Sandwich (try it
with barbeque sauce); Grilled Chicken Salad Deluxe (with light
vinaigrette dressing and your own whole-grain crackers or bread for
carbohydrate); or a small hamburger.

Chick-Fil-A: CharGrilled Chicken Garden Salad (with no-oil salad
dressing) is a smart choice, as is the CharGrilled Chicken Deluxe
Sandwich without mayonnaise and the Hearty Breast of Chicken

Soup with a side salad with no-oil dressing.

Taco Bell: Order a Grilled Chicken or Grilled Steak Taco. You may also order a Bean Burrito, but it has an extra five grams of fat.

Boston Market: Don't think "safe" here, even though this spot gives a sense of healthier fast food. The best choices are the Quarter Chicken (without skin), the BBQ Chicken (without skin), or the Skinless Rotisserie Turkey Breast served with low-fat new potatoes and green beans, steamed vegetables, or zucchini marinara. The best sandwiches are the Turkey Breast Sandwich or Chicken Sandwich, both with no cheese or sauce, with fruit salad or low-fat steamed vegetables. A great main-dish soup is their Chicken Chili; have it with fruit salad.

Kentucky Fried Chicken (KFC): Tender Roast Breast of Chicken without skin, with green beans or Mean Greens. Another choice is the value BBQ chicken sandwich.

Arby's or Rax: Try the Rax Turkey Sandwich (without mayonnaise) or the Rax Roast Beef Sandwich (no sauce). Or try these items from Arby's light menu: Light Grilled Chicken, Light Grilled Chicken Salad, Light Roast Chicken Deluxe, Light Roast Chicken Salad, or Light Roast Turkey Deluxe.

Sub Shops or Delis: Get a small six-inch sub (turkey or roast beef, no oil or mayo). Subway's Roasted Chicken on whole wheat, Tuna with light mayo, Seafood and Crab with light mayonnaise, or the Subway Club on wheat are also good choices.

Pizza Places: Order the personal-size pizza, with vegetable toppings if desired. Eat only half the pizza and save the remaining half for another meal. Or, if you're sharing the pizza with others, try a thin-crust cheese pizza (topped with veggies, banana peppers, or chicken, if desired—no sausage or pepperoni). One slice for women, two slices for men.

Ballparks and Arenas: You may not know about all the positive culinary changes that have taken place at the major league ball parks and arenas. Don't worry, you can still warble "Take me out to the ball game" and "Buy me some peanuts and Cracker Jacks," but now you can add, "Buy me some veggie wraps and carrot juice." Lower-fat foods are tentatively establishing a toehold in the major leagues. Some hard-core fans may stick with beer and foot-longs, but others can choose to eat from the smart parts of the food pyramid while cheering on the home team.

For example, at Edison International Field, home to the Anaheim Angels, health-conscious fans can pick three-bean salad over French fries and sausage sandwiches. At the Cleveland Indians' Jacobs Field, garden burgers and turkey breast on whole wheat compete against fried fish, chips, and pepperoni pizza.

Of course, not all ballparks are into soy burgers and granola. At the Toronto Blue Jays' SkyDome, McDonald's serves as the main food vendor. And a typical SkyDome dessert is funnel cake—deep-fried dough covered with confectioner's sugar. But for the most part, the new foods are catching on—Subway is there providing their low-fat-on-multigrain-roll subs, and salads with grilled chicken are standard. Water—even sparkling spring varieties—is sold right next to flowing beer.

Your eat-smart strategy is not to go into the stands starving and parched, but to top off the tank before you go—and go for the best choices you can while you're there.

APPETIZERS

Many restaurants specialize in appetizers: fried cheese; nachos; fried potato skins loaded with bacon, sour cream, and cheese; fried zucchini and mushrooms; those gigantic onion "blossoms." These are cardiovascular nightmares when you consider that two potato skins or two pieces of fried cheese are basically the fat calories of a whole meal (and should be used as such). Many restaurants are offering raw vegetable platters, but the dip will negate the value of the veggies. If you indulge, do so very carefully.

Smart choices: chicken burritos or fajitas; grilled seafood; marinated chicken breast; non-creamed soup.

BREAKFAST

Breakfast can be a special meal out because most restaurants offer safe and easy choices. If breakfast is later than normal, energize with a snack when you arise, then the later meal. You also may choose to have your larger lunch portions for breakfast and a smaller lunch three to four hours later. Follow these guidelines in ordering:

- Order whole-wheat toast or grits unbuttered; then add one teaspoon of butter, if desired.
- Ordering à la carte is usually safer so that you are not tempted by the abundance of food in the "breakfast specials" or buffets.
- Be bold and creative in ordering. Rather than accepting French toast with syrup and bacon, ask for it prepared with whole-wheat bread, no syrup, and a side of fresh berries or fruit instead. Some restaurants will substitute cottage cheese or one egg for the meat. Many also serve oatmeal and cereal even though it's not always on the menu. It's a nice carbohydrate with milk and fresh fruit, especially strawberries or blueberries.
- Always look for a protein and a carbohydrate source. A Danish doesn't do it!

Smart choices: Eggs scrambled (without fat), or egg substitute, and whole wheat toast or English muffin; French toast (with whole wheat bread) and berries; fresh vegetable and egg-white omelet and toast; whole-grain cereal with skim milk and fruit; Fresh fruit bowl with cottage cheese and whole wheat toast.

Smart Weigh Snacks

Your best eat-smart snack strategy is to keep wisely prepared power snacks wherever you are. Human nature is such that if the right food isn't available, we're apt to reach for the wrong thing—or push through on fumes with no fuel at all. Instead, keep power snacks in your desk drawer, briefcase, or suitcase (refer to the power snack suggestions on page 41).

SMART SUBSTITUTIONS

Instead of...	Choose...
Snickers bar *(280 calories, 14 grams fat, 6 grams protein)*	Crisp apple, mozzarella string cheese *(115 calories, 4 grams fat, 7 grams protein)*
1.74 ounces bag peanut M & M's *(250 calories, 13 grams fat, 5 grams protein)*	2 whole-wheat Wasa crisp breads with 8 ounces Stonyfield Farm nonfat yogurt *(270 calories, 1 gram fat, 12 grams protein)*
60 Ruffles potato chips *(560 calories, 35 grams fat, 7 grams protein)*	24 Baked Lays potato crisps, 1 ounce part-skim cheddar cheese *(300 calories, 6 grams fat, 11 grams protein)*
16 ounces Coca-Cola Classic, 6 Ritz crackers *(299 calories, 5 grams fat, 2 grams protein)*	Bottle of water; turkey sandwich with 1 slice bread, $\frac{1}{4}$-pound turkey, lettuce, tomato, mustard *(214 calories, 5 grams fat, 24 grams protein)*
4 cups microwave popcorn, 1 bottle Snapple Iced Tea *(240 calories, 7 grams fat,) 3 grams protein*	4 cups light microwave popcorn, tall Starbucks Frappuccino *(248 calories, 4 grams fat, 6 grams protein)*
1 jelly doughnut *(220 calories, 9 grams fat, 4 grams protein)*	$\frac{1}{2}$ whole-grain bagel with 2 tbsp light cream cheese, 1 teaspoons all fruit jam *(141 calories, 4 grams fat, 8 grams protein)*
Wendy's medium Frosty *(440 calories, 11 grams fat, 11 grams protein)*	$\frac{1}{2}$ cup vanilla yogurt and fresh berries sprinkled with $\frac{1}{4}$ cup low-fat granola *(205 calories, 1 gram fat, 6 grams protein)*

If the best-laid plans fail and you find yourself face-to-face with the vending machine, wondering which buttons to push, think of this chart below—and go for the tasty, easy-to-find, low-fat yet high-voltage alternatives to all your favorite "sure-to-burn-out-quick" treats.

Traveling the Smart Weigh

Traveling is stressful and depleting in the best of times—even if you're on your way to a week in the sunny Caribbean. And for the road warrior—

the one who does business "by air"—there seems to be no end to travel. While your friends and neighbors might think your job is glamorous, we both know its exhausting. It's not unusual to arrive at your destination dehydrated, drained, and disoriented—surely unfit to be productive or even to have fun. This is especially the case when traveling by air.

Flying causes anxiety. So does rushing to the airport at the last minute, unloading those bags, and lugging that briefcase. Try to arrive at the airport with enough time to relax for a few minutes. Give yourself (and the ticket counter staff) adequate time to get you checked in and your luggage safely on board.

Use these tips to help keep you in tip-top shape—energized, strong, and healthy—for the rest of the trip.

Drink Up

Water, that is. Flying is dehydrating; the pressurized cabin air is ten times more arid than the desert, causing you to lose fluid through your skin. This leads to puffy hands and ankles, fatigue, and a bloated feeling. So drink lots of water—the suggested eight glasses a day plus an additional eight to twelve ounces for each hour in the air. And limit your consumption of alcohol on planes; it is a major dehydrator and has more impact in the air than on the ground. So when the flight attendant asks what you want to drink, ask for water.

Jet Fuel for Jet Travel

Whether a business traveler or a vacationer, you want to be bright-eyed when you arrive at your destination. So don't forget to maintain good nutrition while you're traveling. To short-circuit the stress sequence that accompanies you on your trip, eat adequate pre-flight complex carbs (some whole-wheat bread, cereal, or a banana) with low-fat proteins. Moderate your intake of refined carbohydrates and sugars before and during the trip. Eat more protein and low-fat fare (low-fat dairy products, grilled meats, eggs) to boost your alertness.

On travel days, try not to go more than three hours without a healthy meal or snack. Carry a few convenient power snacks (like trail mix or dried fruit with Laughing Cow Lite Wedges) in your briefcase or purse. While everybody else is eating salted peanuts, you'll be stoking your own furnace with protein and good calories.

Pack some power snacks to keep you on track once you arrive at your destination, too. Eating on some kind of an even schedule will necessitate having your own power snacks available—enabling you to eat the right foods at the right time regardless of where you find yourself during the day. Power snacks will help you accomplish "smart eating on the move" and will keep your stressed and lagging metabolism burning high. Pack foods that don't need refrigeration, such as the trail mix or dried fruits and cheese mentioned above. I take along boxed milk as well.

Airport and airline food can do real damage to your energy and your plan to eat The Smart Weigh. Stay away from caffeine in colas and coffee, and don't get trapped by the high-fat, spicy, and sweet foods throughout the airport. Generally it's wise to order a special meal for air travel (give your airline twenty-four hours' notice). Diabetic meals are highest in protein, fiber, and freshness, and you can enjoy them at no extra cost.

Car Travel

When you drive to your destination, don't be seduced into stopping at the first fast food restaurant or stockpiling a bunch of high-fat, high-sugar snacks when you stop for gas. Surprise everyone—maybe even yourself—by bringing along a bag of healthy snacks. Also make brief stops to stretch, exercise, and breathe deeply so you arrive relaxed rather than stiff and bloated.

Rub in Relaxation

During the trip, put your fingers to your shoulder muscles or temple, and massage. If it hurts, it probably means your muscles are tight. If you're flying, use some of the flight time to relax your muscles and to breathe deeply. You'll arrive at your destination that much more rested. If you are at an exit row or by the aisle, use the space to stretch your legs and do some ankle rotations.

Stay in Shape

How many times have you packed your workout clothes but never made it to the hotel's spa or gym? What about those times you attended a conference at a beachfront hotel or golf course, but you never set foot outdoors once the meetings started? At the very least, plan on a brisk walk each day during your stay, and make time to use the pool or exercise room. You'll be surprised how changing into workout clothes, taking a walk, and breathing deeply will recharge you for the next event or meeting.

Even if you're sightseeing, and are beat from all the walking, you'll still receive an energy and metabolic boost from a focused ten-minute walk that doesn't have you stopping for traffic or great buys.

Give Yourself a Break

Resist the temptation to schedule every moment with activities and people. Leave some quiet time in which to be recharged and revitalized without interruptions. Just a ten-minute timeout—even a power nap—in the middle of your day can restore your alertness and enhance performance.

Finally, Sleep

Road warriors probably know the inside of hotels better than their travel agents. Though there is nothing like your own bed, try to get the same number of hours' sleep at the hotel as you usually get at home. If there's room in your luggage, packing your own pillow will give you a better chance of good shut-eye. And don't use that room minibar for a nightcap as you unwind at day's end. Watch out for those chocolate mints and sweet amenities hotels like to give as your good-night kiss, too.

Time Zone Blues

Jet lag is more than just a sense of being tired; it is an actual discrepancy in the body's intrinsic biological sleep cycle, or "circadian rhythm." Your body's sleep cycle is controlled by the daily alternating sunlight and darkness patterns you experience. When you travel to a new time zone, your circadian rhythm remains on its original biological schedule for several days, so your body's internal clock and the external clock are saying two different things. Your body is telling you to sleep in the middle of the afternoon or turn on in the middle of the night.

Symptoms of time zone blues are fatigue, insomnia, headaches, indigestion, disorientation, and metabolic slowdown, adding up to a serious drain on your enjoyment—not to mention your body's natural ability to process the food you eat efficiently.

Here are some anti-jet lag tips to help reduce the strain:

- Get plenty of sleep during the days and weeks before traveling across time zones, or when daylight-saving time begins (the first Sunday in April) and ends (the last Sunday in October). Starting your trip fully rested will ease the transition.

- Change your bedtime three nights before you depart. If you're traveling west, go to bed one hour later for each time zone difference you experience (up to three hours). If you're traveling east, do the opposite: start going to bed one hour earlier for each time zone (again, up to three hours). Limit your intake of stimulants such as caffeine and alcohol, particularly three hours before you plan to go to bed.

- Get into the day/night cycle of the time zone you're going to as quickly as possible after you arrive. Don't hide in dark museums or hotel rooms upon arrival at your destination—stay out in the daylight. Light acts as a powerful cue to your body, telling your internal clock where you are and what schedule to keep. So does exercise. When you fly east, attempt to exercise at least thirty minutes in the morning sun. When you fly west, attempt to exercise at least thirty minutes in the late afternoon sun. This is one time to resist napping; instead try to keep moving during the day and go to bed in the evening.

- Be careful with sleep medications; they don't resolve the biological imbalance caused by jet lag. Melatonin supplements can be used to correct circadian disorders, but don't take this hormone without first consulting a doctor, and definitely not for long periods of time. Other than occasional use as an anti-jet lag measure, melatonin taken at the wrong time or in high doses can cause sleepiness, sleep disturbance, and impaired work or driving performance—and it may actually shift circadian rhythms in the wrong direction. Moreover, since the Food and Drug Administration doesn't regulate melatonin and other "dietary supplements" for safety and efficacy, there are no standards for purity or dosages.

Don't be discouraged and think you can't ever eat out or travel healthfully. You can have healthy meals away from home; it's just a matter of learning to make good choices. The trick is to learn what you can eat, and then follow through. Rather than feeling dismayed or overwhelmed about everything on a menu that doesn't fit into eating The Smart Weigh, use your creativity and knowledge to find good things that do.

CHAPTER 12

THE SMART WEIGH BINGE-RECOVERY PLAN

IT ALL STARTED AT THE TEX MEX Café: Baskets of crispy fried tortilla chips with melted cheese and salsa, followed by two Texas-sized burritos with creamy guacamole and sour cream. After dinner, she stopped by Krispy Kreme for a donut—or two. And then, since she'd already blown it, she finished off the Oreos while packing the kid's lunches.

The next morning, she averted her eyes from the mirror and pulled out her elastic-waist black pants, mentally chiding herself:

Weakling! Food addict! How could I have been so bad? We tell our kids to say no to drugs, but I can't even say no to a donut! And I had been doing so well—I had been SO on track with my eating and my weight loss. Why did I fall off the wagon—and what's wrong with me?

It's a serious lapse, but even an occasional burrito binge won't make you fat. And it certainly doesn't undo all the good done from living The Smart Weigh in the days and weeks preceding it. The real damage comes from the post-binge hangover. Guilt leads to more overeating and more guilt, and *that's* what leads to the extra pounds. But with a little mental training, a slip-up doesn't have to spell diet disaster. Ditch the guilt and return to The Smart Weigh.

There are physical and emotional reactions you'll need to understand to keep a one-night binge from turning into a week-long slide. Ever notice how ravenous you are the morning after a binge? The culprit is the biochemical gymnastics your body goes through when you overindulge. Your blood sugar swings wildly, triggering an increase in gastric acids, which leads to more hunger—no matter how much you ate the night before. It's enough to make you panic and dive right back into the donut bag or swear off eating for the next few days.

Don't do either, and definitely don't go on a hunger strike! Depriving yourself of fuel throws off your metabolism even further, setting you up for more bingeing.

Expect to feel a little vulnerable the "morning after." Ride it out by calming jittery blood sugars with the The Smart Weigh Binge-Recovery Plan: Strategically eat mini-meals every two hours, balanced between whole-grain carbs and low-fat protein, and get moving. Exercise will equalize the brain chemicals and help process excess insulin.

Make a Plan

One of the worst parts of the food hangover is that helpless feeling that the binge beast is growling outside your door, just waiting for another chance to strike. Tame it by putting yourself back in control. Take ten minutes the next morning to write in a journal just how rotten you feel compared with how good you felt the morning before. Write out your detox eating and exercise plan for the day.

Hide the Scale!

I guarantee you won't like what you see—and it won't be the truth anyway. It's not unusual for an added two to three pounds to show up after a binge—but it's not fat, really. It's just a combination of food and fluid retention from all that fat, sugar, and sodium you took in—and will be higher if you overindulged in booze as well as food. Take at least a three-day break before your next weigh-in—it'll be good for your psyche and will give your body a chance to get back into balance.

Drink Water, Drink Water, Drink Water!

Rather than rushing to the scale to check how much damage you've done, go get a glass of water. And another. And another. Keep downing water throughout the day. Water is a great way to get rid of the extra pounds—it's a natural diuretic. That's why The Smart Weigh Binge-Recovery Plan for "the day after" starts by drinking warm water with lemon. Warm water is less shocking to your system, and the citric acid jump-starts your digestion to finish processing last night's dinner. Keep drinking water all day—the classic advice of eight 8-ounce glasses doesn't apply here; make it sixteen ounces after meals and twelve after snacks. It'll do wonders for relieving your food hangover!

Don't Let the Lapse Become a Collapse

When temptation strikes, think twice before you bite. In your down in the dumps "morning after" phase, it might seem perfectly reasonable to polish off that leftover birthday cake. The lapse becomes another lapse, and before you know it—it's a collapse! Before you give in, remember that emotions can be just as powerful an eating trigger as real hunger, and it's often hard to tell which is which. If you're helplessly craving more, take a 10-minute "time-out" to examine your feelings: Are you really just bored, tired, angry, or lonely? If emotions are fueling your hunger, try a healthy alternative first, like a quick walk. Chances are it will calm you enough that you won't need to eat.

Serve Up Some Self-Esteem

You could spend the next day (or the next week!) berating yourself.

But letting one weak moment cast a shadow over the rest of your life is counterproductive and just plain wrong. You might have *made* a mistake, but you *aren't* a mistake—and it doesn't mean you won't ever get the weight off.

Up Your Calorie Burn—With a Nap!

Sleep is the secret agent of the weight-management game. And more than likely, the binge resulted in a bad night of rest—which further increases stress hormones in the body. This makes your blood sugars fluctuate even more wildly, leaving you hungry and staggering out on a hunt for more high-fat comfort goodies. Even a fifteen-minute nap or quiet rest will do more good than the punitive three-hour gym session you were planning.

Which leads to...

Work Out, But Not Till You Pass Out!

We all know that "I'll just work it off" game, where you calculate your calorie total and vow to pay the price in sweat. But you'd have to spend the whole day at the gym to burn off a 4,000-calorie nightmare. That kind of thinking sets you up to fail—and binge again. You definitely should exercise the next day, but don't punish yourself. Stick with a light cardiovascular workout, like walking and jogging. Think of the exercise as a tension reducer and a way to get back in touch with your body rather than the price you have to pay for being "bad."

The best way to bring a binge to its knees? Again, don't starve yourself the next day! Instead, try eating the following smaller, balanced meals evenly distributed throughout your day—for three days. You'll notice this is the same strategy used to "Jump-start Your Life, The Smart Weigh" in Chapter 2. That's because whether you're doing the program for the first time, or climbing back on the proverbial bicycle after falling off, your body's needs are the same. For sample meal plans for the full three days, refer back to page 28.

The Smart Weigh Binge-Recovery Plan

The moment you are vertical—Drink 8 ounces of warm water with lemon, then a 6-ounce glass of white grape juice to jump-start your hungover blood sugar and quell gastric acids.

8 A.M.—Breakfast of 1 slice whole-grain toast topped with 2 ounces of melted, low-fat cheese, and 1 small banana

10 A.M.—Power shake made with ½ cup frozen berries blended with 8 ounces of skim or soy milk, a dash of vanilla and 1 Tbs. each of oat bran, wheat germ, and ground flaxseed.

Noon—1 sliced orange as an appetizer, 1 turkey tortilla roll (2 ounces of turkey rolled into 1 whole-wheat, fat-free tortilla, spread with Dijon mustard, with shredded lettuce and tomato), plus cut-up raw veggies to munch on.

2 P.M.—1 apple with 2 ounces of low-fat cheese or soy cheese

4 P.M.—¼ cup Trail Mix (1 Tbs. dry-roasted peanuts or soy nuts, 1 Tbs. sunflower or pumpkin seeds, 2 Tbs. raisins)

6 P.M. —8-ounce glass of V-8 juice as an appetizer, 3 ounces grilled fish or chicken, ½ cup steamed brown rice, 1 cup cooked broccoli or spinach, and a green salad drizzled with low-fat balsamic dressing

Before you get horizontal:—½ cup whole-grain cereal and ½ cup skim or soy milk

Defuse Stress, Defeat Bingeing

Now that you know how to survive a binge, let's talk about how to avoid falling into that trap in the first place. One of the most common factors in bingeing is also one of the most common factors in our everyday lives: stress.

I serve as a wellness and nutrition coach for a number of professional athletes, particularly those on the PGA Tour and in the National Basketball Association and Women's National Basketball Association. I also have an opportunity to work with corporate "athletes," high-on-the-ladder executives who are under similar performance demands and pressure. But I work with many more life athletes—people like you and me with stresses and demands from all of life's arenas: emotional, relational, financial, physical.

Like the pros, we life athletes have an individual "court of life" in which we are expected to perform day-by-day with perfection, endurance, and stamina. Like basketball players, we, too, have daily "fouls" committed against us, and we are continually stepping up to the "line"—flanked by team players and opposing forces alike. We are charging full-steam ahead in life with too much to do and too few resources to do it with. So we become drained emotionally, spiritually, and physically. It's a stressful way to live, and we need a different level of fueling and fitness to rise to the continuous levels of stress.

That's where strategic eating and living comes in, with a focus on timing, balance, and variety. Just as your body is designed to work for you nutritionally, it is also designed to survive, even thrive, amidst the stresses of daily life. As important as it is to identify how stress affects us, learning how to defuse life's stressors is even more critical. For once the body picks up a stress signal and interprets "danger," chemical reactions tell the body to go into a conservation mode. This includes three predictable physical responses that clearly affect the whole being.

1. The Slowdown. The body's metabolism slows, storing excess energy in the fat cells for fight or flight. This metabolic slowdown explains part of the quick weight gain that often accompanies stressful times. The slowdown affects energy as well, throwing a person into the fatigue ditch.

Gastrointestinal function is also hit through increased secretions of gastric acids and improper movement of food stuffs through the digestive tract. This means constipation for some; gastritis, ulceration, diarrhea, spastic colon, or irritable bowel syndrome for others. Those prone to increased acidity often have difficulties "facing food" when stressed; they feel a little queasy at all times and can get trapped in a vicious "the less I eat, the worse I feel, and therefore the less I eat" cycle.

2. The Dip. The blood sugar dips, stimulating an appetite for high-calorie foods that will provide needed energy. As the blood sugars fluctuate, energy and moods drop, but appetite soars. Yes, there is a physical reason for getting tired and cranky in stressful times. And, yes, there's a physical reason for craving M&Ms (compounded with strained emotions asking for food to tranquilize the anxiety— after all, stressed, spelled backward, is desserts).

3. The Bloat. The body retains excess fluids, keeping the system lubricated and hydrated for the survival defense. Blood pools in our muscles and extremities, and we store the fluids in the extra poundage in our abdominal area, making us feel bloated and sluggish.

All in all, a stressed body is a rotten place to live—and for some of us it's a 365-day-a-year residence. Some days we face intense, crisis-oriented stress. But some of us live with a level of day-to-day stress that makes us feel chronically out of control to some degree. Chronic stress takes a particular toll on the body because, although it fluctuates in intensity, it never really goes away.

Strategic eating and drinking, exercise, proper breathing, and adequate rest will enable you to stand strong even with a particularly heavy stress load.

The Value of Eating Well

Strategic eating strengthens our barricades against attack and feeds our stress-fighting army. When it comes to righting the fat-storage mechanism of stress and having all the metabolic burn you want and need, eating the right foods at the right time is the bottom line.

Unfortunately, when stress comes in the front door, wise eating often goes out the window. "Quick and easy" takes precedence over nutritious, and that leads to fatigue. The more fatigued we get, the less we exercise. The less we exercise, the more fatigued—and stressed—we become. Next thing you know, you find yourself ordering burritos with everything at the Tex Mex Café.

Although we know that healthy eating and exercise would make a world of difference, they seem more like time-robbers and add to our already long list of "shoulds." If this sounds familiar, try transforming "shoulds" to "coulds." Take charge of what you can. As the body's metabolism slows, properly timed and balanced eating can gear it up. When the stress chemicals produce more gastric acids, smart eating can neutralize the acids and stabilize digestive function. As the blood sugars fluctuate more wildly, the right foods at the right time can keep them even. When the body retains more fluids, adequate protein and fluid intake helps restore proper fluid balance.

Strategic eating keeps your body actively metabolizing the nutrients you eat. In addition, it energizes you for exercise and allows for more restful sleep, both of which further equip the body to alleviate stress.

The Power of Exercise

Exercise is a sword that cuts away at the negative symptoms of stress—a powerful offensive weapon in the war against stress.

Aerobic exercise simulates the physical exertion in the fight-or-flight chemical reactions that occur in the body under stress. It prompts the release of endorphins, powerful stress-busting chemicals. Working somewhat like morphine, endorphins tell the body that it is no longer in danger. You defeated or outran the grizzly bear! You took control of the challenging situation; it no longer controls you.

When you hit a tennis ball, your body thinks you've had your fight. When you walk, your body thinks you are fleeing your present danger; ballroom dancing tells your body that you're waltzing away from the threat. Even laughing is an exercise that contains great stress-busting power—it tells your body that the stress is nothing to fret about. It can't be life-threatening if you can laugh.

Nothing can replace exercise; it is the key to a positive response to stress. This is why exercise is considered nature's best tranquilizer.

Exercise just thirty minutes—it can even become your quiet time in the midst of a busy life, a time when you can see the stress through a different lens.

Ironically, when life is most stressful, when we have the least amount of time to exercise, rest and reflect, eat well, or find anything to laugh about, is when we need those things most. Taking charge of our bodies is one thing within our control, even in the midst of situations that feel very out of control. We can respond as victims or victors.

Think Positive

Weakling! Food addict! How could I have been so bad? We tell our kids to say no to drugs, but I can't even say no to a donut! And I had been doing so well—I had been SO on track with my eating and my weight loss. Why did I fall off the wagon—and what's wrong with me?

What's wrong with me? Bingeing can often be traced to a lack of self-esteem. If you don't feel good about yourself, you're particularly vulnerable to overeating. There's a reason they call them "comfort foods."

A positive mental attitude is a vital spoke in the wheel of wellness—and critical in successful weight loss. In contrast, a negative attitude saps our well-being and aims us toward just what we expect: the worst.

There is both spiritual and scientific wisdom behind having a positive attitude; it is imperative that we set our eyes and our belief on the good things of life. The wisdom behind this is that our mind is a magnet and we gravitate toward what we think about most. We move straight toward whatever we have our eyes on.

Have you ever noticed how often automobile wrecks involve telephone poles? When a car is running off the road, there is much more open space to go toward than there are poles to hit. Yet they are what the driver sees, and they are what the driver hits.

If I continually grouse that nothing ever works for me, that there is never enough time, that nobody cares for me, that only tough things come my way, then I will attract more of the same. Because my eyes see only what I *don't* have, I will overlook opportunity, refuse offers of help, and continue to propel myself into emotional and spiritual bankruptcy.

I have observed that if a person consistently concentrates on what he doesn't have, he will get less and less of what he wants. If we focus on what's wrong, we never find what's right. Alternately, the people who are continually rejoicing in what life gives them, and are always looking for and expecting the best, lead active and fulfilling lives. Those who have the most beautiful lives are those who value life highly.

I'm not suggesting that all the answers to life's problems come simply through "the power of positive thinking," but I do believe that a positive perception goes beyond our circumstances. True joy stems from deep within our souls and flows from our spiritual connection.

Attitude Lifters

Pessimists blame every setback on their personal flaws or on how rottenly the world treats them, and they feel that nothing they do can make it better. It's a state of mind with huge metabolic impact. The negative "I'm gonna go eat worms," or, to be more precise, donuts, response weakens the immune system and locks down the metabolism. Happiness and success—even in weight loss—will be elusive.

Cultivating a positive, optimistic attitude—the belief that you can take charge of your choices and influence your circumstances—protects you against sagging spirits and a lagging metabolism by protecting you against the stress hormones that accompany hopelessness. Try these ten tips to bolster your self-image, lift up your attitude, and keep bingeing at bay:

1. Pay Attention to Your Self-Talk. A negative perspective and negative self-talk become a habitual thought pattern, and it's a hard habit to shake—particularly when it's focused on our own body image. We can be our own worst enemy or our own best friend. It's all revealed in how we talk to ourselves. It's amazing how often we put ourselves down throughout the day—and it's time to stop! We need to replace the negative thoughts with positive ones. It's much like giving our mind and soul a healthy dose of garden Weed and Feed—weeding out the negative belief system, and feeding the one that allows us to thrive.

Next time you catch yourself making critical comments, fight back by immediately complimenting yourself and marveling at how specially you were created. Turn a phrase like, "No one could like anyone as fat as I am," into a positive statement like, "I am liked and respected by others because of who I am. Beauty is an inner quality that comes from caring about myself and about others, not from my weight on the scale."

You may choose to eat well and exercise, but it will not make you a more wonderful, likable person. And believing that you already are that wonderful, likable person is what begins the process of lasting change.

2. See the World Realistically. It's common to compare ourselves to people in magazines or movies, but this is almost guaranteed to make us feel inferior. Realize that envy is a mental state with no payoff. It is human nature to feel sure that others are happier than you are. But the better you know the people you envy—whether the wealthy, the famous, the celebrities with gorgeous partners—the more you will realize their facades hide the same worries, hassles, and sadnesses we all face.

If you must compare yourself to others, look at the real people around you. They come in different shapes and sizes, and none of them is airbrushed or highlighted. Rather than studying pictures in magazines or listening to celebrity talk, read articles or books about uplifting subjects that can raise your spirits.

3. Recognize Your Special Qualities. Make a list of all your positive qualities, not including your physical traits. Are you kind? Artistic? Honest? Good in business? Do you make people laugh? Post your list near the mirror or some place where you'll see it every day.

4. Put Your Body Back Together. Most of us with negative body images have dissected our bodies into good and bad parts. "I hate my thighs and bottom." "My backside is okay, but my stomach is fat and my arms are flabby." Reconnect with your body by appreciating how it all works to keep you going. Try a daily routine of stretching; the fluid movements are great for getting in touch with your body that is so wonderfully made.

5. Remember the Kid Inside You. Give yourself permission not to be perfect. Inside all of us is the kid we used to be—the kid who didn't have to be perfect and worry about everything (or shouldn't have had to!). Give yourself a break. Place a photo of yourself as a child in your bedroom or at your desk at work so you can see it each day and remember to nurture yourself and laugh a little. Spend time with children as well—they are wonderful reminders of how playful and fun life should be.

6. Pepper Your Days With Small Pleasures. Big changes won't make you positive or happy permanently. Negative, unhappy people who win the lottery are no happier a year after they win. But every little thing you enjoy gives you an immediate mood boost. Example: Walk in the park, concentrate on a hobby, or take time off to spend an afternoon with your kids.

One step toward being kind to your body, and inevitably yourself, is to indulge yourself with healthy pleasures. Get a massage, take a long, hot bath, use lotions that smell good, treat yourself to a manicure or a pedicure or go hit some golf balls. It makes a positive statement to your inner self—that you're worth it!

7. Enjoy Your Food. Eating Is Pleasurable. So enjoy it! Food gives us energy and sustains life. Don't deprive yourself or consider eating an evil act. Don't make any food a "forbidden fruit." Focusing on what you shouldn't do and what you shouldn't eat only sets you up for failure. The negative behavior or food becomes an obsession— and it's only a matter of time before you fall headfirst! If you allow yourself to enjoy food, and eat more often, you'll be less likely to overeat. And your body won't feel bloated and uncomfortable.

8. Think Yourself Happier. When a bad mood overcomes us, a slip-up becomes a life sentence of being no good; a bad hair day becomes an "I've always been so ugly" week.

The good news is that it's possible to reverse this negative outlook by becoming aware of it and working to change it. The next time something happens that puts you into a funk, make a mental list of what's going right. You didn't get that desperately needed raise? Oh well, you have lots of friends, and your boyfriend and your dog love you. If a friend forgets to call you at an appointed time, don't be bitter or stay mad. Replace the negative thoughts with happier ones like "Maybe he/she had an emergency" or "Everyone forgets."

9. Be Active. Movement and exercise can make you and your body feel terrific! Not only does exercise help boost your mood, it stimulates your muscles, making you feel more alive and connected to your body. Exercise also distracts you from negative feelings and forces you to concentrate on your breathing, stamina, and physical power. By the time you've completed your workout, your negative feelings are likely to be less intense or even replaced by a positive sense of accomplishment.

10. Thrive! Live well—whatever that means for you. Living well according to a strong value system will help you feel better about who you are and how you look. Whenever a problem seems daunting, take action. Define your goal, then plan specific steps to get there. Every "hopeless" situation you turn around this way will make you a more positive person.

You are a unique, amazing person—don't forget it! A healthy, happy life can be yours.

WEEKLY FOOD DIARY

Your Name:_____ **Week Beginning:**_____

MONDAY

Breakfast	Lunch	Dinner	Comments/Exercise
Protein:	Protein:	Protein:	
Complex carb:	Complex carb:	Complex carb:	
Simple carb:	Simple carb:	Simple carb:	
Added fat:	Added fat:	Added fat:	
Snack*:	Snack*:	Snack*:	

❏❏❏❏❏❏❏❏
CHECK YOUR WATER AS YOU DRINK

TUESDAY

Breakfast	Lunch	Dinner	Comments/Exercise
Protein:	Protein:	Protein:	
Complex carb:	Complex carb:	Complex carb:	
Simple carb:	Simple carb:	Simple carb:	
Added fat:	Added fat:	Added fat:	
Snack*:	Snack*:	Snack*:	

❏❏❏❏❏❏❏❏
CHECK YOUR WATER AS YOU DRINK

*Remember to have a carbohydrate and a protein as a power snack.

WEEKLY FOOD DIARY

Your Name:_____ **Week Beginning:**_____

WEDNESDAY

Breakfast	Lunch	Dinner	Comments/Exercise
Protein:	Protein:	Protein:	
Complex carb:	Complex carb:	Complex carb:	
Simple carb:	Simple carb:	Simple carb:	
Added fat:	Added fat:	Added fat:	
Snack*:	Snack*:	Snack*:	

❏❏❏❏❏❏❏❏
CHECK YOUR WATER AS YOU DRINK

THURSDAY

Breakfast	Lunch	Dinner	Comments/Exercise
Protein:	Protein:	Protein:	
Complex carb:	Complex carb:	Complex carb:	
Simple carb:	Simple carb:	Simple carb:	
Added fat:	Added fat:	Added fat:	
Snack*:	Snack*:	Snack*:	

❏❏❏❏❏❏❏❏
CHECK YOUR WATER AS YOU DRINK

*Remember to have a carbohydrate and a protein as a power snack.

WEEKLY FOOD DIARY

Your Name:_____ **Week Beginning:**_____

FRIDAY

Breakfast	Lunch	Dinner	Comments/Exercise
Protein:	Protein:	Protein:	
Complex carb:	Complex carb:	Complex carb:	
Simple carb:	Simple carb:	Simple carb:	
Added fat:	Added fat:	Added fat:	
Snack*:	Snack*:	Snack*:	

❑❑❑❑❑❑❑❑
CHECK YOUR WATER AS YOU DRINK

SATURDAY

Breakfast	Lunch	Dinner	Comments/Exercise
Protein:	Protein:	Protein:	
Complex carb:	Complex carb:	Complex carb:	
Simple carb:	Simple carb:	Simple carb:	
Added fat:	Added fat:	Added fat:	
Snack*:	Snack*:	Snack*:	

❑❑❑❑❑❑❑❑
CHECK YOUR WATER AS YOU DRINK

*Remember to have a carbohydrate and a protein as a power snack.

WEEKLY FOOD DIARY

Your Name:_____ **Week Beginning:**_____

SUNDAY

Breakfast	Lunch	Dinner	Comments/Exercise
Protein:	Protein:	Protein:	
Complex carb:	Complex carb:	Complex carb:	
Simple carb:	Simple carb:	Simple carb:	
Added fat:	Added fat:	Added fat:	
Snack*:	Snack*:	Snack*:	

☐☐☐☐☐☐☐☐
CHECK YOUR WATER AS YOU DRINK

*Remember to have a carbohydrate and a protein as a power snack.

Weekly Comments:_____

_____

_____

_____

_____

_____

_____

_____

_____

_____

INDEX